To have courage for whatever comes in life
—everything lies in that.
ST. TERESA OF AVILA

For Sue, Jon, and Jenny,
the true and pure gifts of my life

All Scripture citations throughout this book are from *St. Joseph Edition of the New American Bible* (New York: Catholic Book Publishing Company, 1992).

Some passages written by the author and included in this book first appeared in much shorter and different versions in the periodicals *Living Faith*, published by Creative Communications for the Parish, and the *St. Louis Review*, the newspaper of the Archdiocese of St. Louis, Missouri.

Second printing 2010

TWENTY-THIRD PUBLICATIONS
A Division of Bayard
One Montauk Avenue, Suite 200
New London, CT 06320
(860) 437-3012 or (800) 321-0411
www.23rdpublications.com

ISBN 978-1-58595-785-9
Library of Congress Catalog Card Number: 2010920814
Printed in the U.S.A.

Contents

Acknowledgments

Thanks, first of all, to Sue Givens—my first and best critic and editor. I wouldn't be where I am today as a writer and a man if not for her.

Thanks to my family and friends who have supported me with unending prayers as I face my disease and its challenges. You are too numerous to name and too loving and faithful to fathom.

Thanks to my friend Gloria, who suggested I might have this book in me.

Thanks to my editor at Twenty-Third Publications, Paul Pennick, my sometime lunch companion with the Second Thursday Lunch Club. And hey to Bernadette, Teresa, Tom, and the rest of the gang.

Much gratitude to those songwriters who readily and graciously gave permission to use portions of their lyrics—Carrie Newcomer, Tom Kimmel, Kyle Matthews, and my own collaborator, Phil Cooper.

Introduction

That One Word

*You enter the forest at the darkest point, here there is no
path. Where there is a way or a path, it is someone else's
path. You are not on your own path. If you follow someone
else's way, you are not going to realize your potential.*

JOSEPH CAMPBELL

The moment when I got the news from my oncologist is one
of those moments etched in time. If you've ever received similar news,
which is very probable since you're reading this, you know what I
mean. The words tumbled out of her mouth ever so cinematically and
slowly. I think I only heard bits and pieces at first...

Blood disease...very rare...we'll need to do some research...run a
few more tests...don't know for sure what the...

And then it all hit home with the utterance of one word: chemotherapy. Everything snapped into focus. I knew what that meant! Or
at least I thought I did. A million thoughts flooded my mind in a matter of seconds. How would my life be changed? How would I change?
Was I on a fast course toward an early death at forty-seven? Would I

get sick, lose my hair, miss time at work? Would I die, or would this be a blip on the radar screen of my life? Was this just "one of those things" that so many people go through and come out the other end whole and better and changed? What would I tell my wife and kids? Those were the questions I asked myself in that brief moment as I sat on the examination table in an ill-fitting gown.

That one moment—and that one word—was the beginning of a new chapter in my life, to be sure, and one that would change me in many ways. For now, almost three years and two long rounds of chemotherapy later, that change has been mostly positive and life-affirming. It hasn't come without its challenges, of course. There have been times of pain, sickness, confusion, and sadness. But it has also been a time of renewal and rebirth spiritually, and that's the reason I decided to write this book.

Admittedly, my journey through this disease and its treatment, which is often worse than the disease itself, has not been as devastating for me as it is, so often, for others. Perhaps that's the biggest blessing of all. For although many have a story to tell, they are not always able to do so because of the toll their disease has taken on them. So, while I can't compare my experience to those who have fought more aggressive diseases such as cancer or leukemia, I do, at least, have an inkling of what they have gone through. And I know that my own journey is not yet over. I've already had several periods of remission followed by a recurrence, and I know this disease will never fully go away.

I think a brotherhood and a sisterhood exist between those who have battled a chronic disease or undergone chemotherapy or other types of treatment. We are kin, of sorts, those of us who have sat in the recliner or lain in the bed while toxic chemicals were injected into our bodies to try and save us or give us more time. We know each other's pain and numbness and exhaustion. We smile at each other when we meet in the hallways or while blood is drawn, because we can relate and because we know.

Many people have asked how I coped with it all. My initial reply may always sound a bit smug, but it's truthful: I coped because I had no choice. One day I thought I was basically healthy, and the next day someone was scheduling my chemotherapy treatments. This is now just part of my life, as it is part of yours. We accept it as we do a new family member.

But how we accept it all is up to us. I have chosen the way of faith and God because I know of no other way that brings peace and gives me a reason to go on. I know that not everyone shares this view of life and eternity, and I respect that. But I cannot imagine any other view for myself, especially as I grapple with issues of life and death.

So I have opted to embrace my disease and its treatment because I really have no other choice. But I have chosen, as a matter of faith and survival, not to embrace it alone, because my arms are not big enough or strong enough for the battle. However, as I hope you will see in the pages that follow, the arms of my God are big enough to encircle both me and the disease that is attacking me. Whatever the outcome, I have decided to live (and someday to die) held in the arms of God. I can't think of a better way.

To some extent my own story doesn't matter, and as I have written above, I can't begin to compare it to the experiences of others (perhaps you) who have fought tougher and more courageous battles. But on the other hand, you have every right to know a little about me if you're going to follow my journey in these pages. You will get to know me and some of my family and friends in the pages that follow, but for now here's a synopsis of the health issues that brought me to this moment in my life.

In the fall of 2006, I began to experience some painful skin rashes and open sores in several areas, as well as a strange collection of bumps on my scalp. I wrote it off for months as a simple dermatological problem that would eventually go away. But after several different dermatologists and numerous kinds of antibiotics, I still hadn't gotten any better. Finally, the last (and smartest, obviously) of the series of dermatologists decided to do a biopsy, and I was given a preliminary diagnosis of Langerhan's cell histiocytosis (LCH), a rare blood disease that affects only about one in 560,000 adults. Sadly, it's a disease that affects children much more often. Still, it's referred to as an "orphan disease," because it affects so few people and thus very little medical research is carried out on it. As I told my friends and family, "I've always liked the idea of being unusual and standing out in a crowd, but this is not what I had in mind!"

Following participation in a dermatological grand rounds (where my rashes were examined by a procession of about fifteen doctors and medical students), the diagnosis was confirmed, and the case was turned over to an oncologist/hematologist. That's when I first heard the word "chemotherapy" and started to get a little scared.

My wife, Sue, was the only person I had told up until this point, but now I faced the reality and the difficulty of telling my two kids and a few close friends, followed by my colleagues at work. Telling Sue and the kids was absolutely the hardest thing I ever had to do, especially when we knew so little about the disease and the prognosis. Sue, a CPA with a brilliant and methodical mind, set to work finding out all she could about the disease and its treatment. I think she was more interested in the details than I was, and it seemed like she knew as much as my doctor did when we met for the first time to discuss treatment.

My daughter Jenny, who was then fifteen (and is now a college freshman studying to become a music teacher), was direct. She asked: "Could you die?" The words cut me to the core—not because she raised the issue of my mortality but because I knew the pain I was causing her at that moment. My son Jon, who was then twenty and away at college, was quieter and more reflective about the whole thing, which is his way. Both of their responses, of course, were valid, authentic, and reflected the differences in their personalities.

The chemotherapy was set to begin as soon as Sue and I returned from a trip to Ireland as chaperons for Jenny's high school choir. On that trip, filled with anxiety about what the future might hold, I received a wonderful, unexpected, and life-giving gift from the girls and the conductor of the choir. I am a composer and lyricist and, unbeknownst to me, a small ensemble of about ten girls had arranged and rehearsed one of my compositions to perform during the concert tour and insisted that I be guest soloist. I wasn't even told about it until the night before the first performance! We performed the song at about a half-dozen different venues, including the majestic St. Patrick's Cathedral in Dublin and the Knock Marian Shrine.

I'm a firm believer in the healing power of music, so the chance to perform with the choir was just what I needed to get my mind off my impending treatment and centered on the peace that I know only God can give. That gift of music was perhaps the first of so many blessings that have come my way from caring, loving friends and—as is sometimes the case—even from complete strangers.

Chemo started the Thursday after we returned—once a week for six weeks at first, and I was only at the treatment center for a couple of hours each time. I also took a steroid called prednisone and some antibiotics. By most comparisons with others fighting cancer or other aggressive diseases, my treatment was fairly mild and didn't produce as many side effects. Still, about ten days after the first treatment I experienced some pretty intense joint pain in my arms, followed by neuropathy in my hands and feet. The pain eventually went away (although it still returns to some extent with each new treatment), but the neuropathy has been a fairly constant companion ever since April 2007. Still, it's more like "something to deal with" than real pain or illness. I could be a lot worse off, I kept telling myself and others.

A week or two later my hair started falling out, especially when I took a shower. I bought a cool, hip hat and waited. My hair quickly got thin and patchy but I never lost it all.

I finished the weekly treatments and transitioned to a six-month maintenance cycle with treatments every three to four weeks. By then the rashes had pretty much gone away and I was feeling pretty good. At the end of the six months, I learned a new word—remission. It meant a break from treatments and a certain, if limited, sense of hope and relief. I also learned that doctors use the word remission instead of "cured" because there's often no way to tell if and when the disease might come back. I took it as a temporary victory and moved on. My hair came back and everybody told me how good I looked.

The only negatives I felt were the unknowns: Will it stay away or will it start creeping back when the treatments stop? Worse yet, will future MRI scans show the presence of the dangerous cells in other places? My skin was a fairly easy organ with which to work, but an occurrence in another, more vital organ could be far more dangerous. The doctor also noted that the disease could leave me more susceptible to tumors and cancers in the future, so I knew in many ways I'd be dealing with this for the rest of my life.

Indeed, about six months later, a few of the rashes began to reappear, and I thought for sure I was headed to treatment again. I went on a men's retreat at my parish and geared up for the next onslaught. I talked about it. I prayed about it. I wrote about it. I went to confession and bawled my eyes out about my sins and weaknesses. But almost as quickly as the rashes started, they went away. Sometimes your body can take care of itself, my oncologist said. Others pointed to the power of prayer. I was thankful for both points of view.

However, less than a year later the rashes were back again and there was no doubt I needed to go back to "Chemoworld," as I had begun to call it. So, as I write this introduction, I have just completed another initial round of treatment and am headed back into maintenance therapy. Currently, it looks like I'll be doing this for a long time. I feel like an old car, getting serviced and ready for another 50,000 miles. But I'm still running, and life is good.

That's my story, or at least part of it. What follows—the stories, the reflections, the prayers, are a more important part of what I want to share with you. I hope you find something in here that helps you, something you can relate to, something that brings you to your knees or makes you laugh or cry or throw up your arms in worship and adoration of the One who made us all. I pray you can come to embrace what is happening, even as it makes you sick and rocks your world. From the depths of Chemoworld, I hope I can help you in some small way to find and see God. He knows you're there. He knows what you're going through. He knows you by name.

This is my faith. This is what I have learned to embrace. And that's where I'll start.

A few last thoughts as you begin:

I have used the masculine "he" throughout the book when referring to God, not because I really believe God is masculine (or feminine) but because that's my own personal tradition and preference. I hope it's not a stumbling stone for you—I certainly don't mean it to be. Some contemporary conventions for dealing with this issue, such as alternating between the masculine and feminine or just using the word God over and over, even when it becomes cumbersome to the reader (and the writer!) seem to be even larger stumbling blocks. So I've settled on this.

At the end of each chapter I've included three recurring kinds of questions (or "prompts") that you can use for quiet reflection, journaling, or good conversation among friends. I hope you find them useful as a starting place for your own personal journey into your disease, treatment, and survival.

Also at the end of each chapter you'll find a short prayer. I'm a believer in short prayers. My favorite is: "Lord, help me. Amen." Again, I offer these prayers as a starting point. Use them however you want. Whether you read each prayer as a punctuation mark to the chapter before you turn out the light, or you use it as the beginning of a time of personal prayer and contemplation, I hope it helps.

1

Embracing the Mystery

True faith has nothing to do with jollying people along. It has everything to do with facing the fact that things may be an utter and total mess, may be on the verge of going to hell in a hand-basket, with the conviction that God is at work in the mess.

MICHAEL HIMES

For some mysterious reason, my body has decided to throw a wrench into my otherwise very good life. Even though I've been basically healthy for a while now, and my treatments haven't overly disrupted my everyday life, this disease and its treatment have changed me in many ways—some of which I may never even realize. And even though my doctors and nurses are wonderful, and I'm surrounded by caring friends and family and all their prayers, there is no doubt that this whole thing encircles and encompasses me. It is, to a great extent, what I have become. It is who I am. Or at least that's how I feel on many days. No one can really say why I have this disease. It is the great and brooding mystery of my life. So I've been thinking a lot lately about mystery.

Shortly after my first chemo treatments began, I remember going to church one Sunday feeling like one of those proverbial horses that have been "rode hard and put up wet." It was not one of my better days. I ached all over. I was listless. I didn't want to move or think or do anything. I certainly wasn't in the mood to put much effort into praying and singing. I really just didn't want to be there. I would have preferred to have stayed in bed.

But since I was already there, I decided to challenge God, who had given me this mysterious disease. (OK, I knew at some deep level that God doesn't give people diseases, but that was beside the point at that moment.) So I prayed something like, "OK, God, hit me with your best shot. Give me one good reason why I should be here today instead of at home curled up in my nice warm bed with the covers pulled over my head."

I knew it was a silly thing to do, but that was just the way I felt that day, and somewhere inside me I knew God would understand. I didn't really think he would respond but, of course, he proceeded to do just that. From the opening song to the Scripture readings to the homily to the communion hymn, I was cut to the quick with the wisdom and the love and the grace of God that day. Every lyric, every prayer, every nugget of Scripture seemed to be spoken and sung for me alone. If not for the power of community around me, I could have been having a conversation with God all by myself. My God, I thought, you are indeed mysterious and, as we all know, you work in mysterious ways.

So I became intrigued by and drawn to the idea that God, all in all, is a mystery. It's a good mystery, of course. God's a huge, divine, holy, sacred mystery, and the power of that mystery fills my life. But God's still a mystery, and I've decided to embrace that. My daily prayer has become, "Surprise me today, Lord. Reveal to me some of the mystery and meaning behind all that's happening to me."

Since then, I've found myself inundated and inebriated with mystery, as well as by a string of confusing emotions like fear, worry, and a few moments of anger. I have had long and good talks with friends and family. And here's what I've figured out so far: This mysterious disease with its equally mysterious treatment will run its course, one way or another. My doctors and nurses are very positive about the prospects of controlling it. So am I. That's my story and I'm stickin' to it.

But I know there's a flip side to that coin, too. None of us, whether we are carrying around a life-threatening disease or not, know the balance of our life. We don't know if we have a day left or decades. And I believe life is just too precious to spend very much time contemplating the end of it. So in the meantime, I've decided to embrace the mystery of the whole thing instead of running scared. I've been pretty good at telling others to "keep the faith" over the years when such things happen to them, so now it's time to follow my own advice.

I'm embracing the wonder of modern medicine and the wisdom of my doctors, along with the frightening notions behind words no one likes to hear or say, like "chemotherapy" and "cancer treatment center." I'm embracing the power of a healing and life-giving evening of good food, music, conversation, and lots of laughter with my very best friends. Especially laughter. I simply refuse to stop laughing, especially at myself.

More than all this and above all else, I'm embracing the mystery of God's presence in my life, delighting and in awe of the fact that he knows me and has called me by name. As my friend Fr. Gary once said to me, "Never forget that Jesus is crazy about you, Steve." That was powerful for me to hear, even though I already thought I knew it. It helped me remember that God is not just "out there," hovering and lingering over us like a zookeeper. God is crazy about us. As much as I am crazy about my wife and kids, God is way crazier about us all. You've got to like that.

My God is a God of mystery, but not because he is removed and distant and uncaring. In the words of author and priest Michael Himes, "God is mystery not because God is so distant but because God is so terribly close."

My God is the God of all I see and touch and feel. He is the God of all that is coursing through my veins—the good and the bad, the disease and the medicine. God counts not only my days but also the ever-diminishing hairs on my head, my footsteps, and my breaths. He is the God of rare blood diseases and cancer centers and chemotherapy. This is my faith, and my faith is in the mystery of God.

Name five things… about God that make him mysterious to you.

Ask yourself… do these mysteries bother me, or can I bring myself to embrace them as part of my understanding of God? How can I do that?

When was the last time… you felt like Jesus was crazy about you?

God, you are a great and mysterious force in my life. Teach me to understand and embrace your mysteries as I walk the path that unfolds before me. Help me to sense you beside me, my constant companion on the journey, rather than spending time worrying about what might or might not happen around the next bend. Engage me in the present, secure in your presence. Amen.

2

In Chemoworld…

Prayer and love are learned in the hour when prayer has become impossible and your heart has turned to stone.

THOMAS MERTON

The moment the elevator door opens on the seventh floor and I enter the treatment center, I feel as if I am in a different world from the one where I spend the rest of my days and nights. It's different for a number of reasons: the place itself, my fellow travelers in treatment, and my own state of mind and spirit. Chemoworld, I like to call it.

The center, although part of a massive, modern, and sprawling medical center in St. Louis' urban and trendy central west end, is generally quiet, and the people around me seem (again, generally) pretty unaffected, at least for a time, by the world outside the walls of the center. The economy may be falling apart, political candidates and parties may be railing against each other, and war may be raging in far-flung regions of the world, but for a few hours none of that matters as much as the battle being fought between life and death in our own bodies. As killer chemicals are sent racing and screaming into our bodies like tiny Kamikaze pilots on a mission, we're in a different world.

I realize that, so far at least, I have been luckier than many in that my treatments are relatively quick affairs. I'm usually in and out within an hour or two and, while the treatments themselves make me weak and achy for a few days, I'm well aware that many others are not as fortunate. All that could change for me tomorrow, of course. For now, though, I am blessed.

But whatever the length and intensity of my time in Chemoworld, it's safe to say I wouldn't wish the experience on anyone. Still, I have tried to make the best of the time as a short period of quiet, introspection, meditation, and prayer. I realize that many of my fellow travelers to Chemoworld find comfort and peace by having a loved one at their side during treatment. That time of intimacy between two people can be extremely valuable and needed. My wife asked me if I wanted her to accompany me, but I have opted to go it alone, partially so that I wouldn't be burdening her with one more obligation (although obviously she doesn't see it that way), but additionally because I enjoy and need the quiet time to think, pray, or read. That's my choice and I realize it's not everyone's, and I also know that my own desire to have her there beside me might change over time and circumstances.

Chemoworld is no day at the beach, and neither is it a monastery or retreat center. For many it is worse than the disease itself. But I have found that it can be a brief respite and time apart. So if I'm not the chattiest of patients with my caregivers and the other patients around me, it's because I have come to appreciate and savor the relative quiet. There's nothing I enjoy better than good conversation, but I'm also not one for small talk. I don't talk much to my barber or the person next to me on an airplane, either. That's just me.

In any case, this whole experience in Chemoworld has been a good reminder of something that I know well but often forget: God calls us—and even encourages us through the example of Jesus—to make time to get away and spend time alone with him. These "desert" experiences are essential for our spiritual growth, and I have found that to be particularly true during the time of illness and treatment. In fact, "desert" or "wilderness" may just be the perfect metaphors for the experience of chemotherapy.

We go into the desert to be cleansed and refreshed. We go into the desert to relocate our center and re-establish our bonds with our inner life and our God who resides there. Many years ago while on a retreat, I learned from a Marianist priest and writer, Quentin Hakenewerth, the importance of slowing and quieting down so we can find our centers. In a graphic of concentric circles, he showed us all the things in our lives that scream at us and demand attention. At the center was our spiritual self, our soul, waiting quietly and patiently for everything else to quiet down so it could speak. We can only hear that most inner part of ourselves when we move away from the world, when we quiet the screaming voices of advertisers and co-workers and even family members, and go off by ourselves to listen to that quiet inner voice. For it is there we hear our true selves, it is there we hear and can understand what God is saying and what it is he might be calling us to do. Listen closely. Can you hear him?

*Name five things...*that scream for your attention and distract you from hearing the voice of God and your own soul.

*Ask yourself...*when and where can I find the time to get away, quiet myself, and learn to listen for these true voices in my life? Could I do it during chemotherapy?

*When was the last time...*you had a clear sense of listening to your soul or the voice of God? What did you hear?

God, take me by the hand as I walk through the wilderness that is this disease and its treatment. Never leave me alone. Lead me to a quiet place and then help me silence both the world around me and the battle for my attention that rages inside my own head. Quiet me, focus me, and allow me to hear the still, small voice that I know to be you speaking to my soul. Help me to see that this is my truest self, and help me to respond to the call that I hear in these special moments. Give me the guidance I need to face this disease with courage and hope. Speak to me today, my Lord and my God, my center and my all. Amen.

3

Grappling with Life's Numb Moments

*There are only two ways to live your life. One is
as though nothing is a miracle. The other is as
though everything is a miracle.*

ALBERT EINSTEIN

Over the course of my treatment, my chemotherapy drugs have caused what is known as "peripheral neuropathy." In short, my hands and feet are numb. My size-ten feet tingle when I walk, which sounds a little like a line from a Broadway musical, but it's far less entertaining. When the neuropathy first kicked in, I kept dropping things (most memorably a full glass of milk all over the kitchen floor) because my sense of touch had changed with the deadening of the nerves in my hands. I learned to laugh while I cleaned up the messes, and my wife learned to never just hand me a drink without asking, "You got it?"

All in all, I guess it's a pretty small price to pay for the unrelenting work these killer-chemicals are doing to beat the disease into remission, so I'm not really complaining. But nevertheless this numbness is a strange and constant reminder of the whole kit and caboodle—disease and treatment rolled into one unique experience.

Mostly I ignore the neuropathy since there's no point in battling it. But there have been moments when I have been tempted to give in to this numbness in my extremities and let it take over the rest of my life. Sometimes it feels like it would be easier to just give up and give in, even when I know that it's not true. Such was the case one day not long ago when I was at church. There I sat, feeling like I'd really rather be home, watching the Cardinals game, putting my tingling feet up on the ottoman and allowing my peripheral neuropathy to ooze in from the edges and take over the rest of my body and soul. I was numb all over—inside and out—and wasn't in the mood to feel much of anything. At that moment I was almost ready to surrender, to throw in the towel and become a victim to the disease. And "victim" was a word I had sworn to myself I would never use when describing myself and my battle with this disease.

So it's a good thing that my faith, however fragile it can be from time to time, doesn't rely on how I feel. For my faith, I believe, takes me further and deeper and closer to the truth than any feelings I might have on any given day.

So instead of walking out of the church, I settled into my pew to see what God might have to say to me on that fine autumn day. The reading (from Wisdom, chapter 9) grabbed me like an old mother cat grabs a newborn kitten—seemingly roughly but actually gently by the scruff of the neck. I sat up straighter and paid closer attention.

"Who can know God's counsel," it began, "or who can conceive what the Lord intends?" I swallowed hard. Who knows, indeed? The lector continued: "For the corruptible body burdens the soul..."

Even as the words about my corruptible body were spoken (for surely, I thought, these words were meant for me alone), I felt the lightening of my burden. At that instant, I recognized my "condition" for what it was—God's will and intention for me, as least for now. As I accepted (and even rejoiced) in that, I felt the numbness lift itself from my soul and mind, even as it stayed on the tips of my fingers and the balls of my feet. The miracle that took place at that moment was all inside me.

Don't get me wrong. I wasn't then and am not now surrendering to the disease; rather, I am surrendering to God and learning what it means to trust and accept his will for my life. I don't yet know how this disease and its treatment fit into the plans God has for me and my life. The disease is well on its way into "remission," which is still a somewhat scary word because it doesn't quite mean the same thing as "cured." But I'll take it.

Our faith in God doesn't deliver us from the evil of physical disease, nor from the violence and hatred ingrained in the world around us. As people of faith we are not immune from anything that might happen to us as human beings living on planet Earth. But God does ask us to accept his intention for our lives and run the remainder of the race with it. God asks us not to be numb to his meaning and presence in our lives. He asks us not to be numb to those around us.

For our lives, I once heard explained at a funeral service, cannot and will not be measured by the dates of our birth and death but rather by the "dash between," that small line of punctuation etched between those two dates that signifies all we are, all we love, all we have accomplished, and all we have given God in return.

That I (or any of us, for that matter) am here at all—living, walking around, making music, and loving friends and family—is a wonder beyond words. That I am known by God, who has a will and an intention for my life, is a miracle beyond my understanding and a grace I can only accept with humility and awe. And I will not be numb to that miracle. I cannot be.

Name five things... about which you may have become numb.

Ask yourself... what will it take to make me feel again about these things?

When was the last time... you experienced a miracle?

God, I surrender my life to you. I place it in your hands. Use me, just as I am with my weaknesses and disease, however you choose. Remove the numbness from my life as you embrace me and call me your own. Make everything about my life a miracle. Amen.

4

Finding God at the Center

During the period of remission between my first and second rounds of chemotherapy, I attended the funeral Mass for the brother of a friend from church. As the Mass ended, the musicians began playing a song I love and know well, and the chorus of the old Quaker hymn flowed over me like a cleansing, refreshing morning shower:

> *No storm can shake my inmost calm,*
> *while to that rock I'm clinging.*
> *Since love is Lord of heaven and earth,*
> *How can I keep from singing?*

As a musician and a singer myself, I have always been drawn to this song for what I guess are obvious reasons. I have always felt a "call" to sing and make music, and this old song always resonated within me. There is nothing, I once thought, that would ever keep me from singing. But I found out over time that that wasn't entirely true. As I experienced some of the tougher days of my disease and treatment, there were times when singing was the last thing I wanted to do. For me, this was one of the more difficult aspects of coping with my disease. It wasn't that I couldn't sing; it was that I just didn't feel like it.

During the days following the funeral, this powerful phrase from the song returned to me again and again: "No storm can shake my inmost calm while to that rock I'm clinging." And even as the disease and the chemotherapy sapped my energy and sucked me into moments of despair and lethargy, even as they began to shake my inmost calm, I began to realize that it wasn't singing or music that gave me strength and life. Rather, it was God who gave me these important gifts. My singing stemmed from my recognition and acceptance of the gifts and the Divine Giver. I realized that in order to sing, in order to live my life to its fullest, God needed to be at the center of all that I am and all that I do. Music—and all the other joys in my life—would then naturally follow.

The life of a person with a life-threatening or life-altering disease can be depressing and it can be terrifying. On good days, when our heads and hearts are in their right places, it can be also be majestic. Our lives can be frightfully ugly and they can be gloriously beautiful. But even when we seem to be in the midst of our lowest and most distressful times, we can choose to focus on the good and on God and his movement in our lives. Every day we have life (joy, giving, and forgiving) and death (pain, evil, and disease) set before us in so many ways. It is up to us to choose which we will follow. It is up to us to decide whether life or death controls the way we live, even if we cannot control whether or not we will live.

Our daily lives—whether we are battling a disease or not—are where we do the work of the kingdom of God and where, at the same time, evil and illness and violence often seem to reign. So it's hard to maintain that inmost calm even during the best of times.

Even if we consider ourselves people of faith and feel like we have a good relationship with God, it's easy to lose our focus from time to time as the storms of the world swirl around us. Sometimes it seems like it would be easier to just give up and call it a day, retreating into our own little lives and places of relative safety. Sometimes we just want to stop singing.

That approach to life can be tempting, especially in the midst of chemotherapy, but God calls very few of us to lives of holy isolation. God calls us, instead, to lives of action and interaction, to lives that allow others to see an inmost calm at work in us and wonder where they might find such peace for themselves. I made a decision soon after I was diagnosed with my disease and before I really knew the prognosis. I decided that I would do my best to show others that this faith that I had been talking and writing and singing about for years was real and alive and burning within me. I never wanted them to doubt their own faith—or their journey toward God—because of something they saw me do or heard me say.

I tell you about this decision not to brag or claim superiority in any way, for I can't profess that I have always successfully lived out this decision. We all have days when faith doesn't seem to make sense, and others when—try as we may—we are just not very good examples of Jesus and his call to love. Nevertheless, this decision was important and I believe it helped me cope with the day-to-day struggles of living with a disease. My mantra has been: "Let them see Christ…Let them see Christ…even if I stumble and fall."

God calls us to bring Christ and his peace to a world that very often cannot see him or know anything akin to peace because it is spinning out of control and has lost its focus and center. And that's what this idea of finding our own personal center is really all about. As children of God and members of the universal body of Christ, our call is to a life centered on the stability and peace that only Jesus can deliver.

The image that comes to my mind is that of a whirling ballet dancer, spinning furiously but always under control, always spotting that one unmoving point at the top of her spin, where for the briefest stutter of a moment she trains her eyes on something out in front of her and so knows where she is in her spin. She keeps her balance and her center because she is focused not on the spin or on herself but on something beyond herself.

As people of the Word, as church, as people who draw strength from a communal and sacramental life, we, too, have this fixed point, a solid unmoving rock held in the upraised hands of our priests as they proclaim, "This is my Body. This is my Blood."

This is our faith. This is more love and grace than we can fathom. This is more strength that we can muster on our own. This is where we fix our eyes. How can we keep from singing?

Name five things... that distract you and keep Christ from being the center of your life.

Ask yourself... what can I do...what can I pray...to place Christ at the center of my life?

When was the last time... you were able to focus on Christ alone and felt as if he were at the center of all that you are?

*C*hrist, I feel pulled in all directions. I feel distracted by my disease, *by my treatment and by the responsibilities of my life. Center me in your love, O Lord. Be that one unmoving point in my ever-changing life. Be the place where I go when all else seems out of whack. Be the place of my inmost calm. Be my rock. Be the reason for the song of my life. Amen.*

5

Making Sure of God

"Pooh!" Piglet whispered.
"Yes, Piglet?"
"Nothing," said Piglet, taking Pooh's paw.
"I just wanted to be sure of you."

A.A. MILNE

On a visit a few years ago to St. Louis' Cathedral Basilica for a midday Mass, I pushed open the massive doors, and the chilly fall wind behind me seemed to almost blow me inside. "Get in there right now," I could almost hear God say in the gust.

As my eyes adjusted to the dimly lit sanctuary, I saw a scattered body of twenty or thirty devout souls who had made their way here from their jobs, their classes, and their lives. I was not a regular like many of them no doubt were, but I did come here occasionally for holy days or, more to the point on this given day, when it seemed like I should. This particular day was the tenth anniversary of my father's death.

I slid into a pew, removed my coat and tried to breathe normally. I closed my eyes, soaking in the quiet of the stone walls and the linger-

26

ing aroma of spent incense. In some ways, I didn't want to be there at all because, when it came right down to it, I was angry. I'm always angry when I try to figure out what happened to my father's life. His was a life of promise, creativity, and healing cut short by alcohol, cigarettes, and depression. I wanted God's undivided attention on this point. I wanted to scream and pound my fists on his chest like a bewildered child. That not really being an option, I instead lowered the kneeler and dropped to my knees.

At that instant, I remembered a moment more than ten years earlier, kneeling on the cold, tiled floor beside the hospital bed where my father was dying, trying to get on his eye level, trying to make contact with a man who was not all that communicative even in his healthier days. I desperately wanted to see into his mind and soul, to get answers to questions, to get a glimpse of understanding about him and his life. I knelt down because I loved him, even if I didn't understand him. I knelt down because I wanted to be seen by him, and I wanted him to hear the words I whispered. I wanted to look into his eyes and know he was there.

I guess, in many ways, that has been my prayer to my heavenly Father since the day I learned of my disease. I want to know that God is there. I have to know for sure that there is a larger purpose and force in my life. I require something or someone to be sure of, even as I am not sure at all of my own life. I need to know I am not alone.

Thinking back on that day at the cathedral, I remember falling into the well-known rhythm of the liturgy. And like I still do now, on occasion, when I find my mind wandering away from the prayers and toward the aches and pains of my latest chemo treatment, I found comfort in what my body and soul knows and loves best—the blessed gift of the Eucharist, this coming together of the Body and Blood of Christ as both a mystical transformation of bread and wine and a people gathered to pray and be Christ for one another. Even when I am not really fully present and participating, there is a power in this act of communion that refreshes and sustains me. Today, more than ever, I need the power of Christ's Body and Blood in my life, especially as I do battle with my own body and blood.

That day in the cathedral, as my mind wandered to my father, the words of the priest echoed around the cathedral and brought me back: "This is the Lamb of God who takes away the sins of the world. Happy are those who are called to his supper."

And I prayed harder and more earnestly than ever, tears welling in my eyes because my own weakly voiced reply rang so true to me at that moment: "Lord, I am not worthy to receive you, but only say the word and I shall be healed." I was brought to my knees—metaphorically and in reality—as I tried to fathom the immensity of the undeserved and unearned love in which I was about to participate. I was healed.

That day—and many times since—I looked the crucified Jesus in the eyes, stretched to the limit on the cross, Lamb of God and Son of God, blood streaming down his forehead and congealing at his wrists and feet, broken and dying. And I whispered, "Abba. Father. Daddy. I'm not worthy. But I need to know you're there."

Haven't we all, at one point or another in our often confusing and heart-wrenching cycle of disease and treatment, just wanted to make sure we were not alone and that someone was there whom we could grasp, someone who could hear us when we cried out? Haven't we needed to say, "You there, God? I just need to be sure of you."

Name five things... that help you "be sure" of God in your life.

Ask yourself... what am I doing to find God in the midst of my pain and illness? What more could I be doing?

When was the last time... your prayer, your worship, and your intimacy with God brought you to tears? When was the last time you looked Jesus in the eyes?

Jesus, you who know pain and confusion because you experienced them yourself, help me to have a sure sense of you in my life. Draw me ever closer to you through your precious and powerful word, through the intimacy of worship, and through the sharing of your Body and Blood with your church and its people. Never let me forget the power of that communion. Amen.

6

Restlessness

You made us for yourself, and our heart is restless
until it finds its place of rest in you.

ST. AUGUSTINE

As a person of faith and spiritual being, I admit I am a bit of a restless soul. Over the course of my adult faith life, my most consistent prayer, I think, has been something akin to "what's next, Lord?" I seem to be always looking to the next project, the next writing assignment, the next chance to get away and spend some time in prayer and contemplation, the next meeting to do the essential planning for the next whatever.

I always want to pray more than I do, go to Mass more often, read more good spiritual books, be better to those around me, be more compassionate and caring, listen to better and more inspirational music. Sometimes I succeed in doing these things, and sometimes I fail. I'm a bit frustrating to myself and, no doubt, to countless others around me. Why can't I be happy with where I am and with where

God has led me? Why can't I be content? Why this yearning for more, for better, for what's next?

So when I was diagnosed with this disease, there was a part of me that saw the whole situation as "the next thing." Of course, there was another part of me that saw it as possibly "the last thing." Was this God's ultimate challenge for my life? Was this where all of my life was headed and where it would all end?

Even now, a few years after my diagnosis and a few months into my second round of chemo, there are times when I see this time I'm living in as the beginning of the end, even though my prognosis is very positive at present. But no matter how long I live, I have come to embrace a new sense of time. I think more now about my legacy, about what I will leave the world and about what I will leave my wife and kids. Yet I don't find this to be morose, and I am generally not sad about the whole thing. If I were facing a more serious illness with a more definite and terminal prognosis, perhaps I would feel differently, but I hope not. Whatever happens, this has been a good period of taking stock and putting my priorities in order. It has been a time of drawing closer to God. But I still want more. Always more.

I recently read something that gave me some insight into all this. In his book, *Doing the Truth in Love*, Fr. Michael Himes writes: "At the center of our being is an endlessly nagging sense of, 'Yes, yes, yes, but more.'"

I think that this explains the way I feel most of the time. I have this nagging sense of the need for "more," and it's something I just can't ignore. So how do I get rid of it? How can I get some rest from this nag of a notion in the back of my brain? I could pray for that release, of course, but it turns out that's not really what God has in mind for me.

All this restlessness, it seems, is not my fault. It's all the nagging, confusing, irritating work of the Holy Spirit. It is a gift of the Spirit, a gift that keeps on giving. And, at least for me, having a disease is no excuse for saying "no" to the Holy Spirit.

I received the Holy Spirit at my confirmation, and I have prayed for the Spirit's presence in my life many times over the years. There's an old saying that comes to mind: "Be careful what you ask for because you just might get it." I asked for the Spirit. I asked for its guidance. I thought I might get some peace and understanding, but what I got was restlessness and questions. I got what God wanted me to have. This faith stuff is confusing sometimes.

God made us to be restless. He made us to be wondering and wandering and discontented about our spiritual lives, because he knew this restlessness would push us ever towards him. God knew that, with the help of the Spirit, we wouldn't stop, wouldn't accept the easy way of just meeting obligations and skimming by on the bare minimum of spiritual living. God knew that contentment can be the death of spiritual growth. So when we look death straight in the face, when we do battle with it because of our love of life, when we face the very real possibility that our lives may not be as long as we had hoped they would be, I don't think God relents and tells us that it's OK to stop trying to live the life to which we have been called. Quite the opposite.

For when I come to that near-end-point in my life, as we all must, I hope my faith pushes me to keep asking God, "So, what's next?" I believe I want to be restless, even then. Until God decides the time is right to take me away from this world, I hope and pray that my restless need for more keeps nudging me toward God and his will for my life.

My friend Paul Masek, who founded and leads a dynamic and highly effective youth ministry retreat program for the Archdiocese of St. Louis, has a great way of teaching this idea to those on his retreats. He places a large glass of milk in front of the group and proceeds to pour in a large quantity of chocolate syrup. You can hear the stomachs growling. This syrup, he says, is like the Holy Spirit being poured into our lives on the day of our confirmation. Heads nod.

But then the chocolate syrup just sits there on the bottom of the glass, all quiet and peaceful and brown. Nothing much happens to the milk. Nothing is changed, nothing is good and rich and delicious, Paul explains, until we stir it up. We must stir up the Spirit in our lives. The Holy Spirit is not only the syrup; it's the spoon as well. Restlessness is good. Delicious. Filling.

The kids get it. I'm learning.

Name five things… that you are restless about right now.

Ask yourself… where is the Holy Spirit in my life right now? Dormant or alive and stirred up?

When was the last time… you felt a holy restlessness to do more, be more, want more of God and the Holy Spirit in your life?

God, thank you for the restlessness of the Holy Spirit within me. Continue to stir up the Spirit in my life so that others may see its swirling, ever-moving, and all-encompassing power. Prod me, Lord, to continue my search for "what's next," and do not allow this disease to distract me from doing your will and from living fully the life you have given me. Amen.

7

God Laughs at Our Plans

We know that all things work for good for those who love God,
who are called according to his purpose.

ROMANS 8:28

I love reading biographies of successful, innovative, and creative people. Whether the subject is an innovative inventor, explorer, or scientist or a creative artist, musician, or writer, I find inspiration in reading their life stories and learning how many of them pulled themselves up by their own bootstraps and, Horatio Alger-like, overcame adversity after adversity in pursuit of their dreams. The ideal of the self-made man or woman is as American as apple pie, and it makes for a great story.

Most often, one of the shared characteristics of these great personalities is their focus and drive—their abilities to make plans and to achieve goals. And that's a lesson worth learning, to be sure.

In the days and months since I was diagnosed with my disease, I have spent many hours thinking about my life and my legacy—about what I will leave behind for my family and friends. I think about material things such as property and savings, of course, but I spend more time considering more important and longer-lasting assets, such as memories, our shared faith life, and the lessons, wisdom, and sense of hope I want to pass on to my children and friends.

As a writer, I have ruminated over the question of whether or not I will leave behind anything worth reading, calling often to mind one of Ben Franklin's witticisms: "If you would not be forgotten, as soon as you are dead and rotten, either write things worth reading, or do things worth the writing." Sometimes I worry: Will I have done either?

So every once in a while, I find myself being drawn into a funk over this whole thing, and I ask myself questions like: "What if I can't or don't accomplish what I set out to do? What if I don't even finish this book? What if this disease gets in the way of my dreams? What if all my dreams fall through?

Not long ago, in a book by Jewish storyteller Joel ben Izzy, I read this old Yiddish expression: "People make plans and God laughs." A wide, knowing grin spread across my face, and I started chuckling to myself, because I realized that there might be more wisdom for us people of faith in that short, simple saying than there was in all the biographies that had ever been written.

To be sure, there's nothing inherently wrong in making plans and setting goals. I know I wouldn't get much done without my daily planner and my to-do lists. Also, where would I be without the researchers, physicians, and nurses who set goals for their lives and live them out every day so that people like me can live a better and longer life? Goals are good and planning is essential for most good things in life. But there's more to making plans than scheduling meetings and writing down our hopes and dreams in a big "Plan for Success" workbook.

The folly of human plans (and the reason God laughs at them) is that we so often leave God out of them. Even if we call ourselves followers of Christ, we sometimes think we can accomplish our goals in this life through our own strength, our own creativity, our own persistence, or our own intelligence. We may remember to stop and thank God once we succeed (or we may not), but we're often all too willing to accept the awards and recognition for our accomplishments. It's only human, I guess. The problem is, we're more than just human beings. We are children of God.

I think God laughs at us and our silly human plans not out of spite or power but out of divine parental knowledge that he is God and knows what's best for us better than we do. It's like a five-year-old who screams, "I want ice cream for breakfast, and I want it now!" A good parent won't give in to such tirades and may even have to punish the child for the outburst, but he or she may also go out of earshot of the child and begin laughing hysterically because the request is so predictable yet absurd. Ice cream for breakfast, indeed.

As Christians, we need to draw God into our plans and make sure they are part of his plan for our lives. We need to pray for God's will and guidance, not just present him with a business plan for our success and ask him to "sign off on it." God is not our fairy godfather, nor is he a source of funding for our latest scheme. As we bring God into our plans, our deepest desire should not be for success as we define it but, rather, that God's will be done in our lives. That's the promise of a relationship with God and Jesus—not success, health, wealth, and getting our own way. Ice cream for breakfast, indeed.

So even when we find ourselves confronting and battling the most serious challenges and obstacles we will ever face, this relationship with God should not change. In fact, it cannot change, despite our best efforts to thwart it. Because at the moment when we most want to cry out and command God to give us what we want and think we need, God gently and quietly asks us to place our lives in his hands.

When our plans for ourselves consist solely of earthly desires, including a long and healthy life, a little alarm should go off in the back of our heads. That alarm, if we center our lives on our faith and the overwhelming gifts of the Holy Spirit, should sound something like the still, small—perhaps gently laughing—voice of God reminding us who's in charge.

Name five things... for which you have made plans or set goals.

Ask yourself... where was God when I made these plans? What role did I allow God to play?

When was the last time... you prayed more for God's will than you did for your own desires and needs?

God, the provider and source of all that is necessary in my life, look at me today with the loving, laughing eyes of a parent. Give me the faith to place my entire life in your hands. Help me to set goals and make plans that are in concert with your will and design for my life. When I struggle and hurt, gently remind me that I am not alone and that even the pain is part of the plan. Amen.

8

Walking It Off

They that hope in the Lord will renew their strength,
they will soar with eagles' wings; they will run and not
grow weary, walk and not grow faint.

ISAIAH 40:31

When I was a teenager, I was an athlete in several sports, and I remember well the encouragement of my coaches when I would occasionally get hurt. The most frequent thing I heard was "walk it off." Whether I got hit by a pitch or turned an ankle going up for a rebound, this simple instruction was the common prescription for getting better quickly. Thankfully, and almost miraculously, it most often seemed to do the trick.

Our bodies, especially when we are young and healthy, are incredibly resilient creations. In more recent years, I have watched my son playing soccer and marveled at how quickly he could take a fall or a bad tackle and then, almost immediately, get up and begin sprinting down the field after the ball. It's an amazing body we have been given.

So when we find ourselves faced with new physical obstacles and challenges because of disease and its treatment, it's all the more difficult for us because we can't bounce back quite as quickly as we once could. But lately, as my body permits, I have begun to walk. Sometimes I walk across the large college campus where I work. Sometimes I walk around the neighborhood or find an easy walking trail in a nearby park. Sometimes I just walk around the block.

Although I've not yet convinced myself to be a daily walker, I always return from these walks feeling refreshed and strengthened. For a myriad of reasons, I have become physically lazy over the years, even before my diagnosis and treatment. Now I know that I sometimes use my illness to convince others and myself that I just don't feel like getting any exercise. Quite predictably, no one challenges me on those grounds.

However, deep down inside I know that I am just being lazy. Obviously, there are days when I honestly don't feel well enough to get out and walk, and for many in treatment it's even harder. But I am beginning to discern my weakness and set aside those excuses on days when I know it is my will, and not my disease, that is keeping me inside and on the couch.

Recently, I accompanied my parish youth group on a one-week mission trip to Nicaragua, where we helped build homes and a school. On our first day, near the northern city of Chinendega, we were told that we were going to climb Cerro Negro, a 2,400-foot-high volcano that last erupted about a decade ago. When we arrived at the site, dubbed (jokingly, I hoped) the "black hill of death," I stood in awe of the giant black formation. I wondered, and even doubted, if I could climb to the top along the narrow path among the jagged rocks and boulders, and then make my way down the smooth slope of the other side of the hill that was covered with foot-deep volcanic gravel. I knew, of course, that I had an easy out. I could say that I just didn't feel up to it, and no one would question me. But I decided to go for it.

I thought it might be tough, but I wasn't ready for just how tough it was. I stopped often along the way to catch my breath and gather the strength and will to go on. When I reached the top of the first winding and difficult path and saw that it led to another narrow path that shot straight along the crest of the volcano, my heart fell. I realized how much I still had left to do. But I put one foot in front of the other, I put my head down and I just walked. Eventually, I found myself standing at the highest point of the volcano.

The payoff was great. The views were spectacular, and I got to share the accomplishment with the others in the group. We cheered on those who were still making their way up. We shared stories of the ascent and a simple meal of peanut butter and jelly sandwiches. We took photos of each other rejoicing at our accomplishment. And then we headed down—a joyous descent, sliding and jumping through the loose volcanic gravel in minutes and making the multi-hour ascent a mere memory.

I learned a lot about myself that day. I learned I could do more than I thought I could. I learned the power of "one step at a time," and I remembered my high school coaches' encouragement to get past a little bit of hurt by "walking it off." But for me, this day was about much more than walking or physical strength.

I rediscovered an inner strength that I know comes from God. I reconnected with the idea that we are called to take care of our bodies because they are the temples of the Holy Spirit. I'm not going to become a marathon runner any time soon, but my experience on Cerro Negro, along with the intense physical labor of the rest of the week, awakened in me a need to both push myself a little physically (as my body with its disease will allow, of course), and, more importantly, to learn to call upon God as the source of my strength. Walking, which is a simple and accessible exercise for people of many ages, can still be rough going when you're battling a disease and receiving treatment that plays strange tricks on your body.

So when I just can't do it, or when I am winded or I fall, the greatest blessing is knowing that I have a God who sees me in my weakness, who knows me by name, and who picks me up and carries me the rest of the way. I am not ashamed of my weakness, for it is just an outward sign that there is still healing to be done inside me. The greater weakness, I believe, would be to hold on to the anger that I sometimes feel about being old and sick and out of shape. There's nothing to be gained from that emotion. Instead, I find strength in my weakness, because I know that's when God is closest to me.

With every step I take, whether it's a walk across campus or, perhaps, up another challenging hill, I feel myself being drawn closer and closer to Jesus. After all, he certainly knew what it meant to walk in pain up a hill.

Name five things... that you would like to accomplish.

Ask yourself... what's it going to take—physically and spiritually—to accomplish these things?

When was the last time... you really pushed yourself physically, despite your illness?

God, you know the limits of my body better than I know them myself. You know me inside and out. You know when I sit and when I stand, when I walk and when I run. Give me the wisdom to know what I can and cannot do, and then give me the strength and the courage to pursue whatever goal I set for myself. Help me to call on you as my source of strength, and give me what I need today to do what I need to do, whether that's just making it through a rough day of treatment, taking a walk around the block, or getting over an obstacle that I think is too much for me. Amen.

9

Laughter and Friends

Against the assault of laughter nothing can stand.

MARK TWAIN

⚜

I am spending this weekend at a lake in the Missouri Ozarks with my very best friends, and I know it will be a weekend of good food and drink, lots of music, and deep conversation about everything from faith and family to politics, the state of the world, and the latest books and movies. But most memorably and, perhaps, more importantly than everything else, we will laugh. A lot.

The men in our group—Larry, John, and I—no doubt think we're much funnier than we actually are, but we love to laugh at and with each other and at our stories, jokes, and quick comebacks. The women—Dianne, Karen and my wife, Sue—are much wiser and they just laugh at us, mostly, frequently shaking their heads and rolling their eyes. But this is the group of friends that brings me life and keeps me centered and focused on the most important and meaningful things in life.

There is much research that shows that laughter can, in fact, reduce pain and help the healing process. In his book, *The Healing*

Power of Humor, Allen Klein goes to great length describing research that supports the notion that laughter and playfulness can greatly impact a body's physiological systems, including the nervous, circulatory, endocrine, and immune systems. The Internet is rife with articles relating laughter and humor to increased endorphin levels. One article discusses a research study conducted in California showing that even the anticipation of laughter could raise the endorphin levels by twenty-seven percent. Apparently, it really *is* good to laugh.

Laughter, like tears and sharing the intimate stories of our lives, binds people together. This weekend, this close circle of friends will once again be drawn closer together. It is one of the greatest blessings in my life.

From the beginning of this journey with my disease and treatment, I vowed two things to myself. First, I told myself that I wouldn't allow the disease to come between God and me. I knew there would be days when God, church, and my faith would be the last things I wanted to think about and lean on. I knew there would be times when I would point my fists at the sky, beat on my chest, and lash out at God. I knew these things would happen, but I promised myself that I would never allow the disease to steal my faith and permanently rend my relationship with my Creator, my source of strength and hope.

Second, I vowed that I would not lose my sense of humor or my ability and desire to laugh as much as possible, even in the face of disease and, whenever it comes, death. If I was going to be sick, I decided, or even if I was going to die (as we all must at some point), I wanted to do it in the same way that I tried to live—creatively, joyfully, with a song always ready to be sung and a belly laugh or a comical snort never too far distant. For while we may have no choice in the matter when it comes to the slings and arrows that life hurls at us, we do get to choose our response. I have chosen faith, hope, and laughter. I have chosen to continue to be myself for my family and friends. I hope and pray I can maintain that choice when life gets tougher.

Sitting on the deck overlooking the lake with me, these special, close friends—along with a few other close compatriots—never cease to make me laugh and, thus, seek a more creative and positive view of and response to life, even as we share our concerns, fears, failures, and confusion. We take comfort in our sameness and readily accept and embrace our differences. I don't need and can't endure well-meaning but somber, fatalistic, and legalistic conversation from those who are hell-bent on some version of what they deem to be the truth. Especially right now.

Give me instead nimble minds, hearts, and souls that are open to flowing, unguarded talk around a shared table. Give me giant, uncontrolled guffaws and hoots that make me double over and cry. Give me friends who aren't afraid or embarrassed to laugh at themselves or the situations in which they find themselves. Give me friends with whom I can always be honest and with whom I never have to hold back either tears or laughter for fear of offending. Give me friends who take me as I am.

When I lost most of my hair early on in my first round of chemo, we had a good laugh together because they knew I appreciated that response more than I did pity or sadness. When I lost the feelings in my fingertips and frequently spilled my drinks because I lost my grip, we chuckled and snickered and let the cat lap it up. We decided not to cry over spilt milk, as it were.

Laughter—and the company of good and true friends—I have found over and over again, brings me energy and life and keeps me focused on the good that only God can bring. Laughter seems a better reflection of and response to God's grace and love than does self-pity or sadness. Laughter, like faith, seems like the better choice.

*Name five things...*that really make you laugh.

*Ask yourself...*do I surround myself with people who make me laugh and appreciate the goodness of the life I have? Or am I surrounded by those who bring me down?

*When was the last time...*you laughed until you cried?

*G*od, fill my life with good friends, wonderful food, meaningful conversation, and, most of all, the sound of laughter. You are the source of all joy, so bring more laughter into my life, and allow it to pierce my hard edges and find its home deep within me. Help me to see the humor that is present in my life. Help me to laugh at myself. And when I am at those low points when laughter is just not possible, remind me that laughter will come again. Amen.

10

Finding the Sacred in the Ordinary

*Holy is the dish and drain, the soap and sink, and the cup
and plate, and the warm wool socks, and the cold white
tile, showerheads and good dry towels, and frying eggs
sound like psalms, with bits of salt measured in my palm.
It's all a part of a sacrament as holy as a day is spent.*

CARRIE NEWCOMER

I was driving to work one day last week and, when I was almost to my office, I realized that I didn't remember a thing about the drive. I remembered backing out of my driveway and turning onto the main road that would lead me toward the university, but that's all I remembered. I had been so lost in thought and in the business and busy-ness of my day that I failed to notice anything along the way. No stoplights, no trees, no people, no cars around me. How I arrived safely I'll never know. It was like I was on autopilot. That experience of mindless driving, I thought, is exactly how I so often forge ahead through life, unaware that all around me are signs and moments of God's presence and grace.

It's relatively easy to recognize the things in our lives that we have come to know as holy or sacred. If asked to list these elements of life, many of us would quickly rattle off words like church, Scripture, God, Mass and sacraments. We might even branch out further from these distinctly religious ideas and objects and include words like family, children, grandchildren, and friends. We might even recall those special moments in our lives when God seemed especially close—perhaps standing on the rim of the Grand Canyon, listening to a favorite piece of music, or observing a work of art. We might think of holy days and holidays. We might recall weddings and births and even deaths. Certainly all these experiences can be seen as sacred.

But there is also sacredness in the seemingly ordinary moments of my life that, like my drive to work, all too often pass by in a noisy blur without much notice. These moments can be fleeting and seemingly meaningless, but when we take the time to reflect and allow ourselves to live a more examined inner life, we begin to see that the sacred is all around us.

Take this morning, for example. It's a Saturday following a particularly difficult week of work. I awoke to a quiet house, following a good, long night's sleep. I awoke lying next to my wife, my partner in everything for nearly thirty years, my best friend, the person with whom I most yearn to spend time. Is there anything particularly unusual or extraordinary about this morning? Not really. But is it sacred? Absolutely it is, because I am thinking about it and thanking God for it. I am spending time with the idea. I am making it holy by my act of reflection and acceptance that there is a divine force at work in my life.

Later in the morning, I settle in to begin writing this very chapter. My wife and daughter have left to go to the grocery store to buy the makings for our dinner this evening with our good friends. The quiet of the house and the very act of writing become a time of prayer for me. It has the feeling of a sacrament, of my offering up my time, energy, and talent to God. On the one hand, it's ordinary. After all, I write all the time. I write almost every day for my job at the university. But this time of quiet and reflection, sitting at my very ordinary kitchen table, has been made different by my recognition of God's role in it. It has been made holy because I want it to be and because I realize the presence of God in my writing, just as I recognize the living and real power of God in the sacrament and in the people around me when I gather at my church and celebrate the great gift of the Eucharist.

All of a sudden my quiet is shattered by the arrival home of my wife and daughter from the store. I'm there in the kitchen, so I can't escape. My wife has a lot going on today, too, so I know a request of some sort will be forthcoming. It is. Could I cut up the vegetables for the roast? It's an ordinary request, of course. We have always shared the household chores and responsibilities. So I have a couple of choices here. I could beg off, telling her that I'm on a roll with this chapter and would rather not stop. She would understand and say, yes, keep working. Or I can pay attention to the very words I am writing and accept the invitation to make the ordinary sacred.

I can—and do—go over to the sink, wash the potatoes, and methodically cut them into cubes. While I do that, I listen to the music of one of my favorite singers in the background and enjoy the easy conversation between the three of us. I reflect to myself on the joys of the coming evening and how this meal will contribute to a special time among special friends. I thank God for the wonders of potatoes, sharp knives, clean water, and slow-cooked pork loin. I've made the moment sacred—or perhaps moments like these have been sacred all along and God was waiting for me to recognize them as such. What makes the moment holy is our knowledge of the presence of God.

Later this evening I will again remember the sacred moment of cutting the potatoes, even as we bow our heads with our friends and offer up our thanks for the food, for the day, and for our friendship. We will gather around this very table and once again make something very ordinary something sacred.

Don't get me wrong. I don't live in a constant state of spiritual bliss, always aware that God is in the room with me and that everything I do is part of a grand sacrament of ordinary life. Indeed, a week or a month can go by when I don't feel this (or remember to sense it) at all. But I do believe we are all called to this way of living, and we are, perhaps, especially called to it if we find ourselves facing serious disease and health issues. For when we allow ourselves and our lives to be drawn into the realm of the sacred and the divine, even our pain can take on a semblance of the sacred, and our days of chemotherapy can transform into sacramental moments of sacrifice, prayer, worship, and even grace.

Name five things... that can become sacred in your life by your realization of God's presence in them.

Ask yourself... do I believe that God exists and works in my life, even in the smallest and seemingly most insignificant moments? Do I want to believe this?

When was the last time... you experienced something sacred in an ordinary moment or action?

God, make yourself known to me today by calling my attention to the holy things and people that are all around me. Allow me to live my life aware of your movement and your actions. Help me to see the sacred and the sacramental in even the smallest things I do and in the simplest moments of my day. Amen.

11

Calling on the Holy Spirit

We have never even heard that there is a holy Spirit.

ACTS 19:2

From time to time, I like to reflect on the life and words of Christ by putting myself in the sandals of the early Christians. Here they are, trying to figure out exactly what it means to be church, struggling with their beliefs and doubts about the divinity of Jesus, and probably even fearing what this new faith will do to their lives. In short, in many ways they look a lot like me—maybe a lot like all of us. But in the midst of this experience, in the middle of their doubts and fears, they are told: "Wait, there's more. There's the Holy Spirit." And they reply by basically saying, "the Holy what?"

The truth is, it's easy to forget about the Holy Spirit. The "last of the three" in the Holy Trinity often gets the least of our attention as we cross ourselves and mumble the final few words: "In the name of the Father, and the Son, and the Holy Sp…" God the Father is our creator and source of light and life. He's who we generally think of when we say "God." God's pretty hard to forget. So, too, is Jesus. He's probably easiest to get into our hearts and minds because he's right there on the crucifix in front of our eyes. We've seen the movies and read the book. He was one of us. We can relate.

But the Holy Spirit is tougher to get our mind around. We can ask ourselves questions like: Is the Spirit a ghost? Is it the wind or a dove or a tongue of fire? What does it do? How is it different from our concept of "God"? But none of these queries will get us any closer to understanding the Spirit. For the Spirit must be experienced.

For years I had heard the phrase, "be open to the Spirit," but I'm not sure how well I really understood it. Sometimes I thought that the Holy Spirit was just for people who called themselves "charismatic," for those who wanted a more "emotional" kind of worship or prayer or way of communing with God.

But as I came to spend more and more of my life and time writing about my faith and trying to guide others toward a closer relationship with God through my writing, I began to feel more than ever the presence of the Spirit in my life. I have found myself amazed at how an empty piece of paper or a blank computer screen can fill up with words when I turn my writing over to God and ask for the help of the Spirit. The English words "spirit" and "inspiration" come from the same Latin root, *spiritus*, which means "breath." So, for me, this idea of God breathing his Spirit over me feels right. On so many occasions, usually with a writing deadline staring me in the face, I have found myself with nothing to write about and no energy to get the work done. It is during those times that I turn my writing over to the Spirit, asking not only for inspiration but also for the focus and the mindset to get the work done. In short, the Spirit has become real to me because I have seen the fruit and the gifts of its movement within me.

During the course of my disease and treatment, I think I have drawn even closer to the Spirit, because I have allowed myself to be more open to the experience of the Spirit. Just as when I was writing and needed the Spirit to pull me through a case of writer's block, I have learned to call on and come to trust in the Spirit to pull me through particularly difficult times—times when I was feeling physically weak or sick or times when I was feeling withdrawn from Christ and his church. For the Spirit is also referred to as our "paraclete," our source of comfort and advocacy.

Despite my moments of doubt and even disillusion with God and church, this disease, I think, has helped me grow more comfortable with the power and reality of things that I cannot see. My disease, of course, is invisible to me, even though these rogue white blood cells can be tested for and seen with a microscope. I can watch the drip and flow of the clear chemo meds as they run down the tube and into my arms, but I cannot see where they are going or witness their bloody battle with the disease inside of me. It's an invisible war that is raging, and the only proof I have that the chemo is doing its job is that I am still alive. And I've learned that's enough.

We all struggle with our faith at times, and while struggles can make us stronger, they can also leave us weak if we try to go it alone. We simply wear out when we rely solely on our own ability to "keep the faith." That well-worn phrase can become almost meaningless without a deeper belief and reflection upon the source of our faith. Remember: We are not just keeping the faith in ourselves and our ability to cope (although that's important, too). We are keeping the faith in the Giver of all life and everything that is good. The good news is that God has promised to never give us more than we can handle through the grace and guidance and power of the Holy Spirit and its many gifts. As Catholics, we initially receive the Spirit at our confirmation, but we must learn to constantly pray for the presence of the Spirit and for the strength the Spirit provides, if we are to grow to mature Christianity.

It seems that we sometimes treat the Holy Spirit and the gifts of the Spirit as if they are something we can mess around with when we have the time and the inclination. But the Holy Spirit is not a hobby. The gifts of the Spirit are our tools for our life's work and weapons for life's battles.

I'm ready to work. I'm ready to fight.

Name five things... in your life for which you can ask for help from the Holy Spirit.

Ask yourself... when were the times in my life that I felt most connected to the Spirit or had some strong sense of God's presence?

When was the last time... you called on the power of the Holy Spirit for help?

*H*oly Spirit, I invite you into my life today. I ask you to be a part of me and everything that I do and am. Rain down on me your power and gifts. Give me wisdom, so I can see the truth that is before me. Give me understanding and knowledge, so I can learn new things and recognize your grace in my life. Help me guide others toward God and a life of faith. Give me strength in body and soul, especially when I feel weak. Give me a sincere heart that yearns for you. Give me the ability to recognize the power and majesty of God in my life. Show me your power. Come Holy Spirit! Amen.

12

Falling Down and Getting Back Up

*The greatest glory in living lies not in never falling,
but in rising every time we fall.*

NELSON MANDELA

❧

People with chronic health conditions hear the same questions on a fairly regular basis. We get a lot of "How are you doing?" and "How are you feeling?" Depending on how we're feeling and who's asking the question, our answers usually range from a fairly generic "I'm feeling fine" to perhaps the more truthful "Some days are better than others."

I know that when friends and family members—those who genuinely care about me and my health—ask how I'm doing, they are asking about more than the results of the latest test or the toll that chemo is taking on my body. They are interested in those things, of course, but they are also inquiring into the state of my mind and soul. For it's my soul—my very self—that they know and love. And my answer to those questions is pretty much the same: "Some days are better than others."

The metaphor for all this that has been on my mind lately is about "falling down and getting back up." For when we're battling a disease, we all fall down from time to time—physically, emotionally, and spiritually. Sometimes it's relatively easy to get back up, and sometimes it's nearly impossible. And the getting back up is often as painful as the falling down.

But this is not a pep talk about getting up when you get knocked down, or about dusting yourself off and getting back in the game. I know it's just not always that easy or even possible, and to suggest to anyone facing a life-threatening illness that it is that simple would be trite, insensitive, and perhaps even cruel. But what I do want to share are my thoughts on renewal and healing, especially as they relate to our spiritual lives. For when we fall down physically, something we cannot control, our physical weaknesses often take down our souls at the same time. While we can't control the toll our physical challenges take on our spirit, I think that we can control, at least to some extent, the state of our spiritual lives. Our physical ills might be knocking us on our butts and keeping us in bed, but even from that position we have the opportunity and the sufficient grace to reach out to God. As I recently read in a book about contemplative prayer by Jesuit priest Mark Thibodeaux called *The Armchair Mystic*, there's no such thing as being unsuccessful in reaching God, as long as we try. He writes: "I should do myself a favor and memorize this line: To reach for God is to reach God." That "reaching" effort is ours to make, but God will immediately see our effort and lift us the rest of the way.

A song by Christian songwriter Kyle Matthews called "We Fall Down" tells the story of a weary man who every day passes a monastery. The giant walls and the sanctity of the monastery make his life seem meaningless and small. He wonders what it would be like to live such a holy life, to be well fed and warm, to be sheltered from the world. One day, he meets one of the monks and asks him about his life. The monk describes life inside the cloister with these words: "We fall down and get up. We fall down and we get up. We fall down and get up. And the saints are just the sinners who fall down and get up."

The man decides that his life isn't so bad after all, if even the holy monks struggle and fail as he does. So it is with our faith, perhaps especially when we are facing a health crisis. For our faith as Christians is not about being perfect, but it is about always being true. All too often, we try to equate living a Christian life with living a "perfect life," free from sin and hurt, when the truth of the matter is that, on our own, we are entirely incapable of living such lives. St. Augustine wrote that it is not in our power to live as God desires. So we can and should forget about perfection because that ideal can be crippling when we find out that, in fact, we are not perfect. It's dangerous to measure our spiritual lives against some model of perfection. It can lead to falling down and staying down.

But the blessing of a life lived in faith and in the arms of God is that we can, in fact, fall down and get back up. In our faith in God, in our daily lives, and in our relationships with others, we know there's always a way to begin again. No number of self-help books and, certainly, no amount of money, possessions, or psychobabble can keep faith afloat. That can only be done by God, who both transcends the world and, at the same time, moves and works within our everyday lives of faith.

*Name five things...*that make you stumble and fall.

*Ask yourself...*how often do I call upon God to help me up? Do I have faith that God will lift me up when I fall?

*When was the last time...*you needed to simply pray, "Lift me up, God"?

God, today I reach out for you in confidence, knowing that my small effort brings me fully into your presence. See me where I am today, whether high on a hill or deep in one of life's valleys, and be with me. When I fall and cry out to you, hear me and lift me to your side. Never let me fall into a chasm of spiritual despair so deep that I believe I cannot be heard by you and rescued by your love and grace. Amen.

13

My Perfectly
Imperfect Faith

*In the middle of my life, as the day takes its toll, I come to you
on bended knee, stretch out my hand and lift my soul.*

STEVE GIVENS AND PHIL COOPER

I was kneeling after communion on a recent Sunday after a
Thursday chemo treatment, searching my prayers and my mind for
something a little extra to get me through the week. I was exhausted
and sore. I was tired and a little bit grumpy.

On top of all that, my faith, it seemed, was feeling a little less perfect than usual. I was even wondering, as I do from time to time, why
it is that I continue to come to this altar week after week, even when I
don't feel like it, even when I can't seem to find the love of God in my
life, even when I feel at odds with a certain person or church teaching
or when the latest scandal or division of the body of Christ leaves me
feeling wounded or bewildered. "Why am I here?" I asked God. "Why
do I need to do this?"

The answer came in a song that we all began singing at that very moment that equated our need and desire for God with the very air we breathe.

This simple contemporary hymn was the answer to the question rattling around my head and distracting me from worship. I am Catholic, and I continue to throw myself on the altar of God's love week after week because I must. I am desperate for my God and my Savior because this sacramental meal is as real and necessary for me as the air I breathe and the food I eat.

I'm not perfect and my church, its members, and its lay and clerical leaders are not perfect. We do not come before the altar because we deserve to be there or even because we are obliged to do so. Sure, there are church teachings that state we should be at Mass every week, but in a world where personal and individual freedoms hold so much sway, modern Catholics rarely come to the altar because they are afraid not to. We come not because we are perfect examples of Christianity but because we have been invited. We come because of our imperfections. My God is perfect and this great sacrament is perfect, and I have learned over the years that this core belief can and does trump all my weaknesses and failures, if I will put just a mustard seed's worth of faith in it.

My faith in Christ and his church is akin to the relationship that exists between my wife and me. Remaining married is not simply a choice. For us, it's not just an option or a lifestyle. It is what we committed to do and live, and so it has become the very air we breathe. Neither of us can imagine life without the other, regardless of our faults and imperfections. There is no way to separate us. So we continue to breathe and live and share our lives together.

When I was diagnosed with my disease, I faced one of those moments we all dread and fear. Although I was no stranger to illness and death—I lost my mother when she was only fifty-two, my father in his early sixties, and my brother before he turned fifty—I didn't know how I would react when disease actually came face to face with me. I wondered and feared how my life would change and how the whole ordeal would affect my family.

In the end, I realized that, actually, I didn't have a choice. You don't get asked if you're ready for something like this or not. So, other than staying positive and continuing to turn to God in faith and prayer, I had to just keep doing what I always did. Breathe in; breathe out. Repeat. Go to work; go to church. Love my kids and my wife. Hang out with friends. Breathe in; breathe out. And repeat. That's the way it is. That's the way it goes. Perfect or not, it's all I have.

Too many have given up on the church because it has not proved to be perfect enough for them. It is understandable, of course. Our church, which is the perfect gift of Christ to a broken world, will never be absolutely perfect because its pews and its rectories are filled with imperfect people. There is no doubt that many people have been hurt and confused by the imperfect people who make up our church. And so many of these hurt people have left the church or stopped practicing their faith. If we are looking for perfection in our lives of faith and our church, we are setting ourselves up for failure and "lives of quiet desperation," as Thoreau famously wrote in *Walden*. If we are looking for perfection, we should *all* just leave because it's never going to happen here on earth.

But if we throw our very imperfect souls upon the nourishment and life-giving breath we receive in the holy and perfect presence of Christ in the Eucharist, we can be transformed into beings filled with the hope of Christ and the breath of the Holy Spirit. We can be more than the sum of our fears and our imperfections. That's the power of Christ, and that's the message we need to remember. That's the message we should send to our friends and family members who have been hurt and who have left the church. Come on home. We're not perfect, but we know someone who is.

*Name five things...*that sometimes keep you from praying or worshipping regularly or fully.

*Ask yourself...*what are the most important things in my life? What is as essential as the air I breathe?

*When was the last time...*you felt desperate for God's presence in your life?

God, my rock and my sustainer, be my source of perfection in an all too imperfect world. Draw me to your altar and create in me a sense of urgency and desire for the gift of your Son's precious Body and Blood. Make me as aware of and thankful for your presence as I am for the air I breathe. Help me to not get hung up on the weaknesses of people and institutions and the sinfulness of situations but, rather, confirm in me a deep sense of your perfection and grace. Amen.

14

This Little Light of Mine

*You cannot have a perfect day without helping others
with no thought of getting something in return.*

JOHN WOODEN

When I was about four or five years old, my Sunday school
teacher taught my class the song "This Little Light of Mine," complete
with hand motions. During one verse, we held up our index fingers
(like candles) and then covered them with our other, cupped, hands,
while singing the words: "Hide it under a bushel? No! I'm gonna let it
shine!" It's a simple, childlike version of the parable that Jesus tells in
several of the Gospels: "No one, after lighting a lamp, puts it away in
a cellar nor under a basket, but on the lampstand, so that those who
enter may see the light" (Luke 11:33). It's simple, sure, but I've never
forgotten that song.

I've tried to live my life in service to others and have always sought
to be open about my reasons for wanting to serve. I don't serve others because I'm some sort of beacon of goodness or piety. I don't serve
others out of some sense of guilt. I serve others because I have had the

light of Christ placed in my life, and I want to share that with others. God's light is truth, and it is love, compassion, and service to others. I believe I am called to reflect that light back to the world. I believe I am an instrument and a conduit, not the source of the light.

Now I'm not saying that I spend every spare moment of my life in service to others, nor do I believe that a person's commitment to serve can and should be measured in terms of hours spent volunteering for a good cause or the amount of money donated, even though those aspects of service are essential and part of our call as Christians. I think the true measure of service lies in our ability to put the needs of others before our own. This means, of course, that I've failed perhaps just as often as I have succeeded, maybe more. I have failed by being greedy with my time or, sometimes, by just being lazy, which, I suppose, is really just another form of greed.

So when I was diagnosed with my disease and began my treatment, I had a little talk with myself about being of service to others. I knew that taking care of myself (and thus my family) would be of utmost importance. But because my illness was not debilitating, I also believed strongly that my health situation should not change my commitment to serving others. I didn't commit myself to doing anything out of the ordinary—I just tried to keep doing the same kinds of things I'd always done.

Not long after my diagnosis, I was given the opportunity to accompany my parish's youth group on a service trip to Nicaragua through an organization called "Amigos for Christ" that helps builds houses and entire communities for the poor in one of Latin America's poorest countries. Some good friends were going and encouraged me to go along. I was excited about the possibility of doing such "front line" service work and also about the opportunity of traveling to a third-world country to experience for myself the kind of poverty I had only read about. In the end, however, I had to say no because my chemotherapy had just ended, and, even though the disease seemed to be in remission, I just didn't know for sure how I would feel and where the disease would be when the trip was scheduled, which was six months down the road. I regretted having to say no, and when my friends returned, I both enjoyed and felt envious of their photos and their stories. I wanted to serve in that very real way, and I didn't want my disease to stand in the way or give me an excuse.

A year later, my wish came true. In between my monthly chemo-therapy treatments and, by then, much more aware of my body and its reactions to treatment, I was sitting on a plane with about forty others, heading to Nicaragua for a week of service. I knew we were only going for a week, and I knew we wouldn't change the world that much for the people of the villages where we worked in the northern part of the country. But what I did not know was that—working in the shadow of mountains and volcanoes that loom so large over these villages—I would learn so clearly about the courage and fortitude of a community of people who have been dealt a pretty raw deal in life. I learned that they cared about many of the same things that any of us care about and that, when it comes right down to it, we all need food, warmth, friends, and a place to call home.

I also learned that I was no longer strong enough to carry a ninety-pound bag of cement very far, and that I didn't have the same amount of energy that others had for digging ditches and lugging buckets of concrete and gravel. I learned that there were wonderful young people who gladly stepped forward to take my spot on some of the tough-er chores and that a ten-year-old boy from the village could shovel and carry faster than I could.

I learned that I could play with a young orphaned boy with cere-bral palsy and get absolutely nothing—not even a smile—in return. I learned that I could read Spanish well enough to entertain a group of kids, even if part of the entertainment, I figured out, was them laughing at my poor Spanish skills. I learned that we could play games without having to have a winner and that people have immense pride in a home that they helped build, even if that home was smaller and simpler than my garage.

So, I may not have changed their world in a meaningful way, but I know that together we made a difference, and I know I changed my own life and way of thinking about the world. I know the village is just that much closer to having a new school because forty of us worked for a week lifting and pouring and carrying. I know I made a difference because some kids in a small village in Nicaragua now believe there are people in the United States who know about them and can call them by name. I know I made a difference because I dared to take a risk and change my own world by moving outside my comfort zone.

In the end, it doesn't matter what we do, how much we give or how far we travel to do it. What matters is that we give of ourselves, whether we're healthy and strong twenty-year-olds or a fifty-year-old with a rare blood disease who receives chemotherapy every three weeks.

I may be able to go back next year, or I may not. That doesn't matter. But I'm not going to stop looking beyond myself and my circumstances. That is an effort any of us can make. As Anne Frank once wrote, "How wonderful it is that nobody need wait a single moment before starting to improve the world."

Don't wait a single moment. Find your place. Focus on your strengths instead of your weaknesses. Do what you can instead of wallowing in what you cannot. Respond to the call to serve.

Name five things... you could do right now to respond to someone in need.

Ask yourself... what are my strengths? What do I have to offer? How far am I willing to go?

When was the last time... your risked your own comfort to make a difference in somebody else's life?

*J*esus, you taught that we are to love God with our whole heart, mind, and soul, and that we need to love our neighbors just as much as we love ourselves. Help me to take this simple command to heart, and give me the courage and the opportunity to make a difference in the world around me. Give me the strength to go beyond what I have done before and dare to work in your name in ways and places that are beyond my usual level of comfort. Never let me use my disease as an excuse to not serve you and others. Rather, direct me to the places where my abilities and your love are needed. Allow me to be your light in the world. Amen.

15

It's Time to Clear the Decks

*"Who is there like you, the God who removed
guilt and pardons sin?"*

MICAH 7:18

"Good old Catholic guilt" (or Jewish guilt or Protestant guilt, depending upon the joke or the joke teller) is a staple of stand-up comics and situation comedies; the joke supposedly being that it is guilt that keeps believers "in line" as well as "in the pews." I have laughed myself more than a few times at some of these routines, perhaps because I sometimes see myself in them. Guilt can be a tricky thing, and even the most faith-filled individuals can be funny creatures at times. I love a good joke, and I'm not immune to laughing at myself and my foibles, but, in the end, the humor of Catholic guilt falls far short of the truth.

The rest of the story—and the good news behind our guilt—is that we have a God who sees us in our sin and failures and yet embraces and accepts us as we are. God does not want us to feel guilty, nor does he want us to wallow in our guilt. Rather, God is quick to forgive and remove our guilt, offering in its place a life of joy and freedom from sin. To remain in our guilt is not funny. To remain in our guilt is to not accept the gift of mercy God offers. To remain in guilt is our own fault—not God's and not the church's.

A number of years ago—before I was diagnosed with my disease— I wrote the following little story. It is a parable, of sorts, about the importance of dealing with sin and its accompanying guilt, which might be weighing us down or cluttering our lives with worry. Over the years, I have returned to this story, and it has always served as a healthy reminder that it's important for all of us, once in a while, to "sweep the decks clean."

An autumn's worth of fallen leaves, twigs, and acorns have carpeted the decks surrounding my tiny cabin in the Missouri Ozarks, piling up in large mounds in the corners and creating, possibly, a place for snakes and others critters to lie in wait for some unsuspecting interloper like me. It's time to clear the decks.

I grab a broom and walk out into the crisp November air. It's not cold yet, but it will be very soon. The seasons, like supersonic clockwork, seem to mark my time the older I get, zooming past me and returning with frightening frequency. Wasn't it just a couple of months ago that I was doing this? No, it has been a year, my mind tells me as it races backwards, quickly auditing the days, the weeks, the months, the joys and sorrows of the past twelve months. I need to examine my life and seek forgiveness where necessary, I realize. Like these leaves that need to be swept away, it's been a while since I made the long trek to forgiveness, a long time since I asked forgiveness from God and had the ability to forgive myself and others.

As I begin to sweep, a little nugget of Scripture sneaks into my consciousness and I laugh, surprised as always at the little ways that God and his word insinuate themselves into my life at the oddest and seemingly most insignificant moments. But I guess that's the point of a God who knows me better than I know myself, better than I deserve; a God who calls me by name.

"Get behind me Satan! You are an obstacle to me" (Matthew 16:23). Jesus shouted these words, or something like them, to Peter when his good friend tried to save his life, tried to pull him away from his triumphant entry into Jerusalem and his death on a cross a week later. "Why don't we head out to the hill country," Peter seemed to be saying. "Let's lay low for a while." Jesus would have none of it. And so I begin to sweep away the obstacles in my path, wary of lying serpents.

With each swish and sweep, the leaves fly, and my heart opens up to prayer and an examination of conscience, re-calling the obstacles in my life that separate me from God, that pull me away from him, that put other gods (or de-mons) in his place. After about forty-five minutes, I realize my back is aching and my throat is parched. I look around and see all that is still to be done, especially the large deck that overlooks the lake, the one right beneath the big oak. I can't do this alone, I think. I go inside for a break and a glass of water. I walk to the window to take another look at the unswept deck.

I think of my unswept life, my unconfessed sins. I close my eyes and pray, close to tears. Then I walk outside and pick up my broom, for I know the work is mine to do. As I begin, a swift breeze comes up off the lake and pushes me

back, holding me still like the hands of God cupping my
face and shouting: "here I am!"

The breeze gusts and I continue to sweep, realizing as I
do that the wind is helping me, blowing the leaves off the
back of the deck where they can be burned and forgotten.

Since my diagnosis, I think I have found it easier to seek forgiveness, perhaps because I am more in touch with my own mortality and
physical limitations. Or perhaps because I don't want to leave anything to chance. These days, I want to be on the right side of God. I do
not want to leave any space—created by my own sin and selfishness—
between me and those I love or between me and God. No last-second
deathbed confessions for me. That's pressure I don't need.

So, whether I am actively seeking forgiveness from a friend or family member, reaching out to God from the quiet of my room, or seeking
the grace and forgiveness through the Sacrament of Reconciliation, I
have found it easier to do so since my diagnosis and treatment. I have
found it easier to say, "I'm sorry. Forgive me." It hasn't always been
that way for me. But as I experience the pain, confusion, and doubt
of disease and treatment, I find it easier to reach out and seek reconciliation. I find it easier to uncover the humility required, despite my
pride. I find it easier to seek God's face and grace, despite sometimes
feeling like I don't need it or—perhaps—that I don't deserve it.

This is my story. I realize yours may be different, and I can't begin to dictate your route to forgiveness. That you must discern for
yourself. But I can urge you to take a step in that direction, safe in
the confidence and knowledge that you are never alone on that long
walk back to forgiveness and reconciliation. God is surely there behind you, beside you, and before you, gently drawing you forward,
like a cool fall breeze at your back.

Name five things... about which you feel guilty or need to seek forgiveness from others or from God.

Ask yourself... can I wait to seek forgiveness?

When was the last time... you said you were sorry?

*G*od, thank you for the gift of forgiveness, for your unconditional love and grace that seeks and finds me right where I am—even in the midst of my pain and doubt—complete with all my weaknesses, frailties, and sins. Give me the courage to overcome my pride and the strength to look beyond the layers of worry and guilt that have built up in my life. Help me to seek the forgiveness only you can give. And as you forgive me, put a fire in me that burns to both forgive others and to seek forgiveness from those I have hurt. Show me the power of forgiveness and grace in my life. Amen.

16

Groping for God

"...so that people might seek God, even perhaps grope for him and find him, though indeed he is not far from any one of us."

ACTS 17:27

Many years ago when I was a young adult, some friends and I went on what was to be my first and only spelunking adventure. It took place in an ancient cave beneath the Ozark hills of southern Missouri. We entered the cavern through a small hole on the side of a wooded hill just off the rural highway, shimmying our way through the entrance and discovering on the other side an unbelievable world—illuminated only by our flashlights—of rock formations created over millions of years. I remember how, at one point, we all turned off our flashlights and experienced total, utter darkness. I literally could not see my hand in front of my face and, for a terrifying moment, I imagined what it would be like to have to grope my way out of the cave, inch by inch, not knowing if I would ever see the light of day again.

During our journeys of faith, perhaps especially when our journeys include disease or other physical or mental challenges, we can experience "dark nights of the soul" when God seems nowhere to be found and darkness masks any sense of light, hope, or joy. Even our greatest saints and people of faith, as Mother Teresa famously confessed in her published letters, experienced these puzzling and often desperate times. Her confessional letters revealed that she struggled for decades with the notion that God was not present to her. So if we're feeling this way, especially as we struggle with a life-threatening disease, I think we're in pretty good company.

The really good news about this relationship we have with God is that he doesn't expect anything near perfection from us. God doesn't expect us to build international missionary organizations or find a solution to world hunger. But he does expect us to reach out to him, grope for him, try to find him in the dark. Like the woman who reached out to Jesus in Mark's gospel story in an attempt to touch even the hem of his robe, we are called to make that effort (Mark 5:28).

The mystery and majesty of our relationship with Christ is that he is, in fact, always near, awaiting our groping hands to reach out to him in prayer, seeking forgiveness and yearning for his welcoming touch.

When we reach out to God, we connect in the dark and we seek a kind of healing that can be spiritual, mental, and even physical. The idea of healing is tough to get our head around sometimes, I admit. For if we pray for healing—especially physical healing—what does it say about our God when we do not get better? I don't think it means that the healed person prayed harder or had more faith than the person who remained sick. I don't think God works that way.

A poll conducted by *Time Magazine* in 1996 found that eighty-two percent of all Americans believe in the healing power of personal prayer. A *Newsweek* poll confirmed the findings a year later when seventy-nine percent of respondents said that they pray regularly and that they believe God answers prayers for healing. What those of us who profess these beliefs are telling the world is both fundamental

and monumental: God is not just an idea. God is not just a philoso-
phy. God is not just looking down on us from a distance. Rather, our
God is alive and real and plays an active role in our lives.

What God asks of us in return for his presence in our lives is simple and yet—at times—frightening. God asks that we put all our faith
and trust in him. God doesn't ask that we put some faith in him and
the rest of our faith in our education, the stock market, or the bank. If
we really believe that God gives us everything, then we must learn to
give him all that we have in return.

As a start, we must bring ourselves to make a gesture that shows
that our faith is as real as our God is. Our faith must become a verb,
not just a thing that we set on the shelf or hang on the wall and take
down when we need it during tough times. Our faith must become
a part of everything that we do. The gesture that God asks of us is
simple. We must reach out and touch his cloak. Or, like Peter on the
stormy Sea of Galilee, we must step out of the boat, take that first
small step, and believe that God will support us when we dare to walk
upon the waves (Matthew 14:22-33).

In Mark's gospel, a father brings his sick son to Jesus to be healed.
Jesus tells the man that his son can be healed if he will just have faith.
To this command the man replies: "I do believe, help my unbelief!"
(Mark 9:24). This simple, honest prayer of a man who wishes Jesus
to heal his son seems to be the essence of all the prayers I have ever
prayed. I do believe, or else I wouldn't be praying, but I know I need
more faith. God understands our need for more faith, just as God understands all of our human weaknesses.

What God requires of his children is neither a perfect theological
faith or even our unwavering belief in his existence and role in our
lives. Rather, God wants us, like the crowds who constantly pushed
around Jesus as he walked from town to town, to come to him with a
small grain of faith and a deep desire for more. We must grasp after

God, hoping to touch the hem of his garment so we might be infused with more faith in God's love and compassion.

Most of us pray, if for nothing else, for the protection of ourselves and our families and friends. For me, my prayer every night for God's protection is my ultimate statement of faith. It says I trust God and place my life in his hands. It says I know that I live only because God allows me to live. It says I know God could demand my life today. It says I know the world is full of anger and disease, and yet I go on because I have faith in God and in the meaning he has given my life. It says, "Here I am, Lord, reaching out for you."

Name five things… in your life that represent that you are reaching out to God, seeking his healing touch.

Ask yourself… do I believe that God can heal me—emotionally, spiritually, and physically?

When was the last time… you felt a prayer had been answered?

*F*ather God, see me here in the darkness of my soul. Give me the wisdom and the strength to reach out for you, to grope for you, to yearn for you and your healing presence. Give me the faith I need to cope with all that life has thrown at me secure in the knowledge that there is no problem so big that I cannot handle it with your healing and grace. More than anything else, help me to seek your will for my life. Amen.

17

If You're Happy and You Know It…

Happiness is when what you think, what you
say, and what you do are in harmony.

MOHANDAS K. GANDHI

❧

More than a few times in the past couple of years, someone at home or work has asked me, "What's wrong?" Obviously, I guess, I wasn't looking very happy or perhaps I was letting out one of my trademark heavy sighs that my wife knows so well. Although I can't always put my finger on exactly what is wrong, it's clear that my unhappiness must be showing.

"Not being happy" is not a crime, of course, especially if you're coping with something like a disease, pain, or the dread of your next chemotherapy treatment. But I also feel strongly that I don't want my particular situation and worries to become any more of a burden than they already are for those I love. I have a strong desire—a call even—to be happy so they can be happy, even if I don't always succeed at that.

To be clear, those closest to me—my wife, my children, and my friends—do not place this expectation of happiness on me. They've never told me to "be happy" or "put my best foot forward." They are all too aware and understanding of the fact that there are going to be times when I'm less than happy. They've seen me unhappy many times and love me just the same. So any pressure is my own. Still, I just don't believe that my disease should give me a free pass to be glum all the time and bring others down with me. I don't want to allow myself that excuse.

Nevertheless, as I recently pondered my periodic unhappiness, I began to wonder if maybe my state of mind and behavior were some kind of sign that I was letting God down on my obligation of being light and "being Christ" for the world to see. I began asking questions like, "Would Christ frown or grumble or complain?" and "Are we called to be happy?" I've been thinking about those questions a lot, and I've come to the conclusion that I've got some work to do on myself.

Over the centuries, philosophers have had much to say about happiness. Aristotle said that happiness could be gained by living virtuously. Rousseau said that happiness came from having a good cook, good digestion, and plenty of money. In some sense and on some level, those old philosophers are probably right. But as Christians, we are called to a much higher level of happiness.

What Jesus says is, "I have told you this so that my joy might be in you and your joy might be complete" (John 15:11). God made us, and God made us to be happy. More importantly and more precisely, God made us to be happy "in him." Other important aspects of our lives (like family, friends, accomplishments, and money) can make us happy for a while, but they can just as likely make us sad or angry. God is much more than just one of the things that gives us joy. God is the source of all joy. God is joy, just as God is love.

Many common sources of joy are temporary. They may make us happy for a moment or a day or even a year, but if they are not from

God, they will only lead to separation from God. Even serious vices, addictions, abuses, and personal failures have the potential to make us happy for a while. There's no doubt that they produce moments and experiences of something akin to joy. But none of those will last, and eventually the vices or failures separate us from God.

As people of faith, we know that God loves us, and we try to love him in return and obey his commandments. Even so, we still may not be happy because of our personal situations or because of our perception of the world and the people around us. So we either blatantly blame others for our unhappiness, or we unconsciously do it, and sometimes we lash out for unrecognizable reasons at the people we most love. But we also know somewhere deep inside that our happiness is our responsibility. Thomas Merton may have said it best: "We are not at peace with others because we are not at peace with ourselves. And we are not at peace with ourselves because we are not at peace with God." It always comes back to God and us.

So as we continue our journey of life that now includes words and ideas like disease, chemotherapy, diagnosis, remission, relapse, hope, and doubt, it's important to remember this simple article of our faith: God loves us. We know God loves us because we can see and feel him moving and working in our lives. All of the blessings we receive—life, family, food, water, nature, music, answered prayers, beauty, talent— they all come from God and are expressions of his love for us.

Being a Christian doesn't mean we will never be sad or angry or depressed. God knows we will struggle, but he still calls us to joy and happiness, and he still wants us to be his face to the world. So I'm choosing, as often as I can, to smile. It's a small thing in the grand scheme of things, I know. But if my smile is authentic and engaging to those around me, and if it, in some way, reflects to the world that my happiness is found in my relationship with God, then it becomes an effective, even contagious way of professing my faith in the face of adversity.

What I seek is a harmony and completeness in my life, a state of mind and soul in concert because I am not conflicted within myself. I seek a state of happiness that comes from knowing that all that I do, think, and say comes from my relationship with God and from my knowledge that he knows me by name and wants me to be filled with his joy.

*Name five things...*that you have done that have made you truly happy.

*Ask yourself...*how often do I take out my unhappiness on those closest to me?

*When was the last time...*you felt that your life had really been changed because you actively chose happiness?

God, I know that I sometimes need to be reminded that joy and happiness really are better than isolating myself in self-imposed pity or misery. I know that sometimes I like to wallow in my own "blues" and take others down with me. So inject me today with your spirit of joy. Give me an authentic smile and a heart filled with the kind of happiness that only you can deliver. Help me be happy, Lord, and help me spread that joy to others. Never allow me to use my health as an excuse to deny joy to myself and those I love. Amen.

18

Being Born Again
(and again and again)

"How precious did that grace appear the hour I first believed."

JOHN NEWTON

⁓❧⁓

A number of years ago, while channel surfing, I saw the renowned American poet Maya Angelou on CSPAN's "Book TV" addressing an audience. I remember watching her for a few minutes and then, right about the time I was ready to surf on, she said something like: "I met a young woman recently who told me she was a Christian. I said to her, 'Already?'"

I grinned and nodded in amused agreement. Her point, of course, was that Christianity, or "becoming a Christian," is something we grow into, something that seeps into us and transforms us over time. I believe it is certainly the most life-changing thing that ever happened to me, but I don't believe it happened in one flashpoint, soul-saving, born-again moment. Some Christians do believe in this sudden transformation. I can't speak for them nor would I argue with them.

They have their own faith stories to tell, as do I, and I realize that God works in many wondrous and grace-filled ways.

This is not to say that I don't believe in the concept of being born again, because I do. Let's review the story from the third chapter of John's gospel. An important member of the Jewish community named Nicodemus comes to Jesus and tries to butter him up by saying, "I know you are a teacher from God, because no one else could do the things that you are doing on their own." Jesus says, basically, "That's right, and no one is going to see God and his kingdom unless he is born again." The guy is confused by this kind of talk, and asks how a grown man can be born again. He talks about the biological impossibilities of this. Jesus explains that a man must be born again of "water and spirit," meaning he should be baptized. He talks about "flesh being flesh" and "spirit being spirit" and tells the man not to be amazed by all the confusing talk. But, of course, Nicodemus is still pretty confused and amazed, and we can't really blame him, can we? So Jesus says, "Wow, you're not all that bright for a guy who's supposed to be so smart. Tell you what, I'll make it simple: just believe what I say and focus on the spiritual stuff" (John 3:1-18, paraphrased).

That story explains what being born again is all about, and Jesus doesn't really get any more specific about how to go about doing that except that we're supposed to believe in him and pay attention to the spiritual stuff of our lives. So that's what I've been trying to do for quite a long time now. Sometimes I think I'm doing OK, but sometimes I struggle with the spiritual stuff because the "flesh stuff" seems to be demanding my attention, especially during these days of disease and treatment. That's a big reason why I think being born again needs to be an ongoing process and a journey back to Christ that continues every day of our lives. It is a choice to be made again and again.

I say I am a Christian, and I profess the faith of the Catholic Church as the foundation for my spiritual life. But, in fact, I think it's truer to say that I am becoming a Christian. For I think we need to be reborn, we need to become like little children, we need to crawl to God on our hands and knees every once in a while and beg for forgiveness and salvation. I think we need to do it over and over again not because it didn't "take" the first time but because we have not yet been perfected, have not yet been made whole and complete. So we continue to be reborn and continue to seek the love and grace of Christ. Through that grace, I have come to experience my rebirth in Christ in so many ways and during many circumstances over the years. Some are monumental and sacramental moments. Others are experiences of the sacred taking place in otherwise ordinary moments, but they are, nonetheless, moments of new life.

I was born again when I was about ten years old, sitting scared and excited and a bit confused in my friend Timmy's church, where his father was a part-time minister. I can feel the weight of the man's hand on my shoulder as he prayed with me and asked me if I believed that Jesus died for my sins.

I was born again a couple of years later at a giant Billy Graham Crusade at the Arena in St. Louis, when I went forward with thousands of others and dedicated myself to Christ.

I was born again as a seventh-grader on the day of my confirmation and first communion at the United Church of Christ where I was baptized and brought up in the Protestant Christian faith. I remember standing proud in front of the congregation and being asked questions by my pastor on the essentials of my faith. I remember taking the strange wafer from the plate and the tiny glass cup filled with grape juice. I knew that what I was doing was important and real, symbolic of the Lord's last supper and of my own adult initiation into the congregation.

I was born again as a seventeen-year-old on a Catholic high school retreat after several years away from a church of any kind, sitting in a small chapel surrounded by images and sounds and smells that I did not understand, but which somehow proclaimed to me that God was present and real.

I was born again on the day I was welcomed into the Catholic Church at age twenty, when I received the chrism of confirmation and the imposition of the Holy Spirit by the Archbishop of St. Louis.

I was born again on the day I married Sue, when we became one with each other and with God, a cord of three strands that cannot be broken.

I was born again (and again) when I witnessed Jon and Jenny being born, miracles of life and love so wondrous that I could not possibly doubt God's hand in it.

I am born again each time I stretch out my hands to receive the Body and Blood of Christ, the true presence of Jesus in my life and in our world.

I am born again at the sound and depth of music that truly moves me—the soaring of Miles Davis' horn, the soul of Dave Brubeck's piano, the comfort of James Taylor's voice and guitar, and the majesty of Yo-Yo Ma's cello.

I am born again standing in front of the colorful impressions of Monet's gardens or in the midst of 50,000 St. Louis Cardinal baseball fans.

I am born again with each sunset I share with Sue and our friends.

I am born again spending precious swaths of time with Jon and Jenny and their friends, mesmerized at the adults they have become or are in the process of becoming.

I am born again standing in the midst of the poverty of a small village in Nicaragua, amazed at how little it takes to have joy and contentment.

I am born again with each short prayer that begins each day, each whispered "amen," each song sung at the top of my lungs, each "thank you, God."

I am born again, right now.

───❧───

Name five things... that can make you feel renewed and reborn.

Ask yourself... how aware have I been of these moments of rebirth? What are the benefits of being more aware?

When was the last time... you felt the revitalizing hand of God on your life?

───❧───

God, I come to you today seeking the kind of new life that only you can give. Allow my faith to become more than mere contentment and, instead, place in my heart a deep desire and yearning to become new with each passing day, to recognize your spirit and life in all that I do and experience. Open my heart to these daily rebirths that shepherd me along on this journey of faith that you have given me to live. Amen.

19

Learning Gratitude

Don't pray when it rains if you don't pray when the sun shines.

SATCHEL PAIGE

The day of my most recent treatment a few weeks ago, Clarice drew my blood perfectly and painlessly. Tammy processed my payment and somehow made me feel OK about it. A nurse's aide whom I had never met before (and whose nametag was flipped so I couldn't see it) took my vitals and didn't snicker at my weight. My regular nurse practitioner, Susan, was on vacation so I got to meet Barb, who was equally attentive. My young oncologist/hematologist, Todd, poked and prodded and asked all the right questions. Misty hit the vein the first time and gave me my push of vinblastine.

If it takes a village to raise a child, it takes a modern hospital (many the size of a small town) to care for a patient like me. I didn't want to be there, of course. I would have preferred to be just about anywhere else. And I really don't like being "cared for" because, like most people, I like to think that I can take care of myself, that I am self-sufficient. By nature, I just don't like to bother people.

Nevertheless, I am learning to be grateful for all of this care. It's something I've been working on, something that doesn't come easily or naturally to me. The truth is, when we're battling a disease or even fighting for our lives, gratitude to others is not always the first thing on our minds. We are centered, as perhaps we need to be at the time, on our own health and recovery.

But, in reality, what I have seen over and over as I have received my treatment is that the vast majority of patients show enormous gratitude for what is taking place around them. Most of the people I meet during my Thursday treatments seem cheerful and at peace with the process, even though I know from my own experiences that they are certainly suffering times of anger and disappointment. They seem thankful to be where they are and appreciative of the mysteries and miracles of modern medicine and the genuinely caring people who deliver their health care.

Our gratitude for the good in our lives begins with our awareness of it. While this may seem obvious, it is also obvious that we all too often cruise through life without stopping to think about such things. When we become genuinely aware of those around us and how they are serving us, our gaze shifts from looking only inward at ourselves and our own challenges to looking outward at the world and the people around us. This shift of perception enables us to consider the great acts of love and service that we receive every day. We stop to think and consider that the technician who draws our blood does the same thing for hundreds of others each week, and so we become thankful for the fact that she is there to perform that essential process for us. And when she gets it wrong and has to poke us a few extra times, as she might on occasion, we are still able to smile and say "thank you" as we offer her our other arm.

As people of faith, as believers in a triune God who is creator, savior, and spiritual light all wrapped up in one, we are called to lives of gratitude and thanksgiving. Our gratitude begins with God as our source of life and everything that is good and beautiful. But Jesus asks us to love God first and love our neighbor as ourselves (Mark 12:30-31). So gratitude that begins and ends with God is not enough, for it does not recognize the kindness, generosity, and service of those around us.

With rare and miraculous exceptions, God does not physically touch us and change our lives. Instead, God has chosen to work through human beings. Christ has given us all the opportunity to be his hands and feet and eyes for the rest of the world. Perhaps this divine calling is nowhere more evident than in those health care workers who care for us and guide us along on our journey toward wholeness and healing.

Besides the dedicated doctors, nurses, and technicians that care for me, I also have come to experience Christ in the actions and the simplest of gestures heaped on me by friends, relatives, and even by people that I don't know at all who have called or written encouraging notes in response to some article or spiritual reflection I wrote about my illness.

At times I feel nearly overwhelmed and consumed by this spirituality of gratitude, by a life filled with the awareness of God and the people that he has placed in my life. The thought that—despite my weaknesses and health challenges—my life is filled with these caring individuals brings me to my knees and nearly to tears of joy and gratitude. The knowledge of God's hand working in concert with their hands draws me as close to God as is humanly possible.

So I have chosen to live a life of gratitude and thanksgiving instead of one of regret and fear. Over and over I know I must choose creativity and joy over self-destruction and anger. I choose life over self-imposed death. I choose love. I choose faith. I choose God.

For the wonderful and gifted health care professionals that God has placed in my life, I offer this beautiful reminder of the power and spirit of God that they represent to the rest of us. It is often attributed to St. Teresa of Avila, but the true source appears to be unknown:

Christ has no body now but yours.
No hands, no feet on earth but yours.
Yours are the eyes through which he looks
with compassion on this world.
Yours are the feet with which he walks to do good.
Yours are the hands with which he blesses all the world.
Christ has no body now on earth but yours.

Name five people…who care for you and for whom you are grateful. Then pray for each of them.

Ask yourself…do I remember to thank them for what they do, and do I remember to thank God for their presence in my life?

When was the last time…you said "thank you" to these people in a meaningful way that showed them how truly grateful you were for them and what they do for you?

God, I come to you today overwhelmed by the thought of all the people you have placed in my life to care for me. From family and friends to nurses and doctors to the strangers who hold doors and offer a smile, I thank you for the richness and authenticity of the love and care I experience every day. Never let me forget that these people are reflections of the pure light and love that emanate from you alone, that they are your hands and feet and eyes for a weary world. Thank you for showing yourself to me in this way—for even my sometimes weak faith can see and understand true grace when it looks me in the eyes. Amen.

20

Emptying Ourselves to Make Room for God

Contemplative prayer in my opinion is nothing else than a close sharing between friends; it means taking time frequently to be alone with him who we know loves us.

ST. TERESA OF AVILA

⟨◈⟩

There's an old story, attributed to the Curé d'Ars (St. John Vianney) that tells about an elderly man who enters his parish church every day, sits for a while in silence, and then leaves. One day the parish priest (the future saint) asks him about what he does every day. The man replies simply: "I look at God, God looks at me, and we enjoy one another." I don't know if I've ever heard a more clear and instructive description of prayer.

I think sometimes we try to make prayer far more difficult and complex than it really is. There is no right way to pray, of course, and what may be fruitful for one person might be as dry as a desert for another. We can say the prayers we learned as children that have been etched into our brains and souls. We can recall or read favorite passages of Scripture or poetry. We can just talk to God about what's going on in our lives. Or, like the old man in the church at Ars, we can just sit with God and enjoy the company.

Many people talk about being "filled" by God while in prayer, and that can be an apt description of what can happen in prayer. But here's the problem: If we're too full of ourselves and our busy lives, there's just no room for God. So we have to empty ourselves.

Perhaps this is all the more important to consider when we are fighting a life-threatening disease or undergoing the rigors of intense treatment like chemotherapy. We are often full of so many emotions like anger, doubt, worry, and fear, as well as the disease-killing chemicals themselves that are making us sick. But even then—perhaps especially then—we need to focus on making some space in our lives where God can dwell within us.

My friend (a pen pal, actually), Sr. Immaculata, is an eighty-nine-year-old Sister of St. Joseph from Sault Ste. Marie in Ontario. She has spent her life in prayer and service, including teaching piano to children, something she still does regularly. In one of her recent notes to me she included this quote from the great mystic, St. Teresa of Avila: "There is no stage of prayer so sublime that it isn't necessary to return often to the beginning." Sr. Immaculata added: "That's where I am right now and very happy to be there as I find the Lord being very gentle with me." At age eighty-nine, she says she needs to "keep working for a closer relationship with God." If she does, certainly the rest of us do, too.

When I was first diagnosed with my disease and began treatment, I felt myself being pulled to the starting point where all prayer begins, "back to the beginning," as St. Teresa writes. Although I continued to pray with words for myself and for my family and friends, the kind of prayer to which I felt most called was less about dialogue with God and more about my sense of God's presence when I prayed. I perceived God reeling me in, drawing me with an invisible yet powerful rope to a closer relationship with him. For returning to the beginning, I think, is about placing ourselves in the presence of God and then making room for him. Like for an old married couple, it's sitting before the fire together that means so much, not the words that are spoken or left unsaid.

Or perhaps a better metaphor is that of a mother and a newborn child. For that intimate relationship is not about words but about presence. It's about the sense of touch and being held. It is about confidence and comfort and warmth, even though the child cannot possibly utter those words.

That's what I want and need from prayer these days. As I settle into my armchair or relax in bed before falling asleep, my most urgent and felt prayer is that I am being seen and held by God. Like Sr. Immaculata, "I find the Lord is being very gentle with me," and I think that's because I am allowing him to be, especially on days when the aches and pains of treatment are consuming me.

I've struggled with prayer in the past. I worried that I was not doing it right, or I was overly concerned that I should be getting more out of it than I perceived I was. I think I was waiting for God to hit me over the head with a two-by-four of divine revelation or give me a Grand Canyon sense of his presence, when all the time I should have been quiet and listening for a still, small voice that was whispering: "here I am."

A few years ago, inspired by the story of St. John Vianney and the old man in the chapel, as well as this growing sense that I needed to empty myself in order to make room for God, I wrote a song called, "Empty Myself."

In the morning as the light breaks
I rise to face another day.
All my worries, all the distance
All the ways I fail to say:
I am filled to the brim.
I am filled to the brim.

In the silence, in your presence
I bring you all I have and hold.
All my loves and all that glitters,
All my gifts and dreams of gold.
I am filled to the brim.
I am filled to the brim.

So I empty myself.
Empty myself. Empty myself.
And I pray, "fill me up."

In the evening as the day fades
I stop and try to find your gaze.
I look at you and you look to me.
I see beyond my mindless haze.
I am filled to the brim.
I am filled to the brim.

So I empty myself.
Empty myself. Empty myself.
And I pray, "fill me up."

*Name five things…*or experiences of prayer that draw you closer to
God.

*Ask yourself…*do I ever take the time to just "be" with God? When
and where does that happen? What do I need to do or rearrange in
my life to experience that more often?

*When was the last time…*you felt embraced by God?

*God, draw me closer to you, and allow me to spend time just held in
your embrace. Give me the words I need to pray to you from my
innermost self, but also give me the serenity and the wisdom to seek and
covet times of silence with you, moments when no words are necessary.
Hold me in that silence. Amen.*

Writing from the
Depths and Dark

There is nothing to writing. All you have to do is
sit down and open up a vein.

RED SMITH

As a writer and as a person who receives chemotherapy on a
regular basis, I think I can relate to what the famed sportswriter Red
Smith is saying here, especially when it comes to writing about my
disease. In short, it isn't easy and it's sometimes painful, but I know
that I must do it, just as I must show up at the treatment center to accept the needle.

Writing down our thoughts, our feelings, our beliefs, our fears, our
joys, etc., can have a therapeutic effect on our minds and souls. The
very act of writing, in fact, can be a prayer, an opportunity to open
ourselves to God as well as to those who might read what we write.

Over the years I have, from time to time, taught creative writing to
adults in a number of settings—from a parish library to a community

center to a correctional facility. The one thing that just about all of my students had in common was this: They thought they didn't have anything to say, nothing worth writing about and no story to tell. That is, until they finally sat down and wrote. When asked, "How do I learn to write?" or "How do I become a writer?" my consistent advice to would-be writers over the years has been: "If you want to learn to write, then you must write." That seems all too simple an instruction, but it is absolutely true. No amount of talking about writing or reading books about writing or taking writing courses will make you a writer. You must commit yourself to sitting down and actually writing. The physical "work" of writing is what makes us writers.

So, when my students finally put pen to paper or fingers to keyboard and allowed themselves to take the "risk" of writing and of being honest with themselves and with their potential readers, they could barely stem the flow of what poured from them. They were truly astonished to find out they had something to say to the world and could, in fact, muster the words to express it.

I think there is something deep in all of us that yearns to tell a story—something in our DNA, perhaps, or something we have inherited as a collective member of the human race. In the days before television and radio, and even before the days of printing, humans gathered around fires and told the stories of their lives. They created myths to try to explain both the wonders and the fears of the world around them. Something in us yearns to tell our story.

You're just about finished reading my story—or at least a part of it, for certainly there's more to my story than this—so perhaps the question you should be asking yourself today is: "Should I tell my story? Should I write it down for myself or my family or maybe even for thousands of people?" I hope you answer yourself with a resounding "Yes!"

But how to get started? That is always the hardest and trickiest part, of course. There's not one answer to that question. If there were, it wouldn't be so hard and tricky, right? Common advice for writers and would-be writers is to keep a journal to record what's happening in their lives, whether that record of their life and experiences is just for themselves, for their family members or future generations, or for a larger, more public audience. I have taught my students the advantages of keeping such a journal, the main one being that it gets them into the habit of writing, hopefully on a daily basis. For many, this form of storytelling comes to them naturally and they take to it like a pig to mud. For others it's drudgery, for they can't imagine why the details of their lives will ever be of interest to anyone else. To be honest, I'm one of those people who have never been able to consistently keep a journal, even though I've tried many times. But there are other ways to get yourself writing.

Many people don't consider themselves writers and yet find it quite easy to write creative, poignant, lengthy letters to old friends and loved ones. Some people can't imagine accumulating twenty or fifty thousand words—enough to fill a book over time—but find it easy to write in shorter spurts and thus are drawn to shorter forms of writing such as poetry, essays, prayers, or reflections. Your writing abilities reflect your call. Write what you can and you are writing what you are called to write. In fact, that holds true in life as well. Do what you can do well, and you are responding to the call of God in your life.

Whatever form your writing takes, keep in mind one characteristic that all good autobiographical writing has in common: When you do it right, it can feel risky. You are risking:

- being honest in order to help someone else understand their own circumstances;

- receiving criticism or doubt from those around you (even those closest to you) in order to tell your story;

- challenging yourself and your faith in order to become stronger;

- being authentic in order to show others your true self, your fears, and your passion for your life, your faith, and your God.

- devoting time to writing (instead of to other things) in order to respond to your call to write.

But it's worth the risk, whether you are writing a book for many to read, a letter that might be treasured in your family for generations, or a poem to be discovered someday by some unknown person on a folded note stuck between the pages of your favorite book.

My friend Tom Kimmel, a gifted and spirit-filled songwriter who lives in Nashville, wrote these words in his beautiful song, "Pages":

You know me by the stories I have made.
You know me, looking out through boxes and cages.
And it's hard to clearly see what's right in ordinary light.
Does the truth filter down through the ages?
We cannot see the end
So here we must begin.
Tell me what will we write on these pages?

Do you feel a calling right now to get a part of your life and experiences down on paper (or on your hard drive)? Then don't hesitate and don't wait. That feeling of being called (or even poked!) is one of the ways that God communicates with us. Respond to that gentle call. Take the risk. Take the plunge. You have story to tell. Tell it.

Name five things (stories, lessons, emotions, beliefs)...about which you could write.

Ask yourself...do I have the courage to write honestly about these things so that I might help others understand what I have been going through, so that I might help them in some way?

When was the last time...you took the risk of putting your real, authentic self out for the world to see?

God, the Creator of all that is good and wonderful, help me to be a creator. Help me reflect a little bit of your light and grace to those around me. Give me the courage to be authentic and honest in my words and actions. Give me the strength to speak and write openly about the challenges that I have faced or am facing so that I might help others face their own challenges. Help me get past the idea that I have nothing to say and no story to tell. Give me the words I need to express my innermost thoughts and my deepest fears and convictions. Allow me to get past the fear. Be my courage. Amen.

Notes

INTRODUCTION

1. Diane K. Osbon, ed., *Reflections on the Art of Living: A Joseph Campbell Companion* (New York: HarperCollins Publishers, Inc., 1991), 22.

2. "LCH in Adults," *Histiocytosis Association of America* (2007), http://www. histio.org/site/c.kiKTL4PQLvF/b.1763811/k.8B13/LCH_in_Adults.htm.

CHAPTER 1

1. Michael J. Himes, *Doing the Truth in Love: Conversations about God, Relationships, and Service* (Mahwah, NJ: Paulist Press, 1995), 140.

2. Ibid, 8.

CHAPTER 2

1. Thomas Merton, *Seeds of Contemplation* (New York: New Directions, 1949), 140.

CHAPTER 3

1. Albert Einstein, as quoted on QuotesDB.com, http://www.quotedb.com/ authors/albert-einstein.

CHAPTER 4

1. Alf McCreary, ed., *St. Patrick's Breastplate* (Belfast: Appletree Press Ltd, 2006), 64-67. The version of the prayer as reprinted in this book is traditionally attributed to C.F. Alexander (1818-1895).

2. Robert Lowry (1826-1899), "My Life Flows On (How Can I Keep From Singing)" as reprinted on Hymnsite.com, http://www.hymnsite.com/fws/hymn.cgi?2212.

CHAPTER 6

1. A.A. Milne, *The Complete Tales of Winnie-the-Pooh* (1926; New York: Dutton Children's Books, 1994), 284.

CHAPTER 6

1. *The Confessions of St. Augustine: Modern English Version* (1977, Grand Rapids: Baker Book House, 2005), 15-16.

2. Himes, 38.

3. Chocolate syrup and Holy Spirit analogy developed by Paul Masek, Coordinator of The REAP Team, A Catholic Youth Retreat Ministry of the Archdiocese of St. Louis. He further develops the concept in his book *Stirring It Up* (St. Louis: Out of the Box Records, 2007).

CHAPTER 7

1. Benjamin Franklin, *Poor Richard's Almanack* (New York: Skyhorse Publishing, Inc., 2007), 68.

2. Joel ben Izzy, *The Beggar King and the Secret of Happiness* (Chapel Hill, NC: Algonquin Books, 2003), 20.

CHAPTER 9

1. Alex Ayres, ed., *The Wit and Wisdom of Mark Twain*, as quoted from "The Mysterious Stranger," ch. 10, 1916 (New York: HarperCollins, 2005), 134.

2. Allen Klein, *The Healing Power of Humor* (New York: Tarcher/Putnam, 1989).

3. "Get Ready to Laugh! Even Anticipating Laughter Raises Endorphin Levels," www.SixWise.com (12 April 2006), http://www.sixwise.com/newsletters/06/04/12/get-ready-to-laugh-even-anticipating-laughter-raises-endorphin-levels.htm.

CHAPTER 10

1. "Holy as a Day is Spent," ©2002, Carrie Newcomer. Used by permission. All rights reserved. From the album *The Gathering of Spirits* on Rounder Records, www.carrienewcomer.com.

CHAPTER 12

1. Nelson Mandela, *Long Walk to Freedom* (1995).

2. Mark E. Thibodeaux, *The Armchair Mystic: Easing into Contemplative Prayer* (Cincinnati: St. Anthony Messenger Press, 2001), 16.

3. "We Fall Down," ©1997 Kyle Matthews, Universal Music MGB Songs/ Above the Rim Music/ASCAP. Used by permission. All rights reserved. From the album *Waking Up to the World*, www.KyleMatthews.com.

CHAPTER 13

1. "After Communion," ©2005 Steve Givens and Phil Cooper. Used by permission. All rights reserved. From the album *Brighter Still* by Nathanael's Creed, Potter's Mark Music, www.nathanaelscreed.com.

2. Henry David Thoreau, *Walden* (Boston: Ticknor and Fields, 1854), 4.

CHAPTER 14

1. John Wooden, *Wooden: A Lifetime of Observations and Reflections On and Off the Court* (Chicago: Contemporary Books, 1997), 10.

2. "This Little Light of Mine," Harry Dixon Loes (1895-1965), public domain.

CHAPTER 16

1. *Time Magazine* and *Newsweek* polls referenced by Winston Morrow in his article "The Power of Prayer" (2003), http://www.alternative-doctor.com/soul_stuff/prayermorrow.htm.

CHAPTER 17

1. Mahatma Gandhi, as quoted by John Cook, comp., *The Book of Positive Quotations* (New York: Random House, 1999), 15.

2. Terence Irwin and Gail Fine, eds., *Aristotle: Selections* (Indianapolis: Hackett Publishing Company, 1995), 350.

3. Jean Jacques Rousseau, French political philosopher (1712-1778), Quotation #1724 from *Laura Moncur's Motivational Quotations*, www.quotationspage.com.

4. Thomas Merton, *The Living Bread* (Toronto: Ambassador Books, 1956), xiii.

CHAPTER 18
1. "Amazing Grace," John Newton (1779), public domain.

CHAPTER 19
1. Leroy [Satchel] Paige interview, *New York Post*, 4 October 1959.

CHAPTER 20
1. St. Teresa of Avila, as quoted in the *Catechism of the Catholic Church*, 2nd ed., s.v., par. 2709.

2. *The Collected Works of St. Teresa of Avila*, trans. Kieran Kavanaugh and Otilio Rodriguez (Washington, DC: ICS Publications, 1976), 94.

CHAPTER 21
1. Walter Wellesley "Red" Smith, as quoted by Ira Berkow, *Red: A Biography of Red Smith* (1986; reprint, Lincoln, NE: First Nebraska Paperback, 2007), 208.

2. "Pages," ©2000 Tom Kimmel and Jenny Yates, WB Music Corp/Drala Music/In My Dreams (ASCAP). Lyrics used by permission. All rights reserved. www.tomkimmel.com.

More Resources *for*
Your **Spiritual Growth**

Beyond Pain • *Job, Jesus, and Joy*
MAUREEN PRATT

This inspiring book is for anyone who lives with deep, life-altering pain and who wants to have more joy, faith, and purpose. It challenges readers to follow the example of Job and most of all Jesus, in accepting pain and in believing there are many joys awaiting them, if they choose to reach out, look, hope, and live…beyond pain.

168 pages • *$14.95* • *978-1-58595-786-6*

With the Dawn Rejoicing • *A Christian Perspective on Pain and Suffering*
MELANNIE SVOBODA, SND

This deeply spiritual exploration of pain offers encouragement for anyone dealing with suffering—whether physical, psychological, or spiritual. It is rooted in Scripture and real life, and its 36 brief chapters touch on the many ways pain affects our lives. Recently diagnosed with a rare autoimmune disorder, Sr. Melannie writes from personal experience and with deep wisdom.

144 pages • *$12.95* • *978-1-58595-699-9*

Sacred Healing • *MRIs, Marigolds, and Miracles*
JANET DAVIS

Each of these recollections encourages readers to find comfort in Scripture and prayer, as well as in the ordinary things of life. They address those who are too sad and overwhelmed to seek companionship with God and others, and offer assurance that sacred healing is possible when they allow God's powerful love to embrace their hurting souls.

216 pages • *$14.95* • *978-1-58595-798-9*

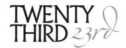

1-800-321-0411 • WWW.23RDPUBLICATIONS.COM